TAKE
CONTROL

---

of your

DIABETES
RISK

TAKE
CONTROL

---

of your

DIABETES
RISK

JOHN WHYTE, MD

CHIEF MEDICAL OFFICER *of* WebMD™

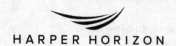

HARPER HORIZON

Take Control of Your Diabetes Risk

Published by Harper Horizon, an imprint of HarperCollins Focus LLC.

Any internet addresses, phone numbers, or company or product information printed in this book are offered as a resource and are not intended in any way to be or to imply an endorsement by Harper Horizon, nor does Harper Horizon vouch for the existence, content, or services of these sites, phone numbers, companies, or products beyond the life of this book.

This book contains advice and information relating to health care. It should be used to supplement rather than replace the advice of your doctor or another trained health professional. If you know or suspect that you or your child has a health problem, it is recommended that you seek your physician's advice before embarking on any medical program or treatment. All efforts have been made to assure the accuracy of the information contained in this book as of the date of publication. The publisher and the author disclaim liability for any medical outcomes that may occur as a result of applying the methods suggested in this book. The author has changed names and identifying details to preserve the privacy of patients and other individuals.

ISBN 978-0-7852-4065-5 (eBook)
ISBN 978-0-7852-4064-8 (HC)
ISBN 978-0-7852-4067-9 (SC)

Library of Congress Control Number: 2021947487

Printed in the United States of America
23 24 25 26 27 LBC 5 4 3 2 1

TO LUKE AND JACK

I love what I do but being your
dad is the best job I could ever have.

An ounce of PREVENTION

is worth a pound of CURE.

—BENJAMIN FRANKLIN

CONTENTS

INTRODUCTION

ARE YOU SURE?

That's the initial response many people have when they are told they have diabetes, or prediabetes. "How can this be happening to me when I don't eat that many sweets?" Or, "I know plenty of people who are less healthy than me and they're fine." Some even argue, "No one in my family has diabetes, so why did I get it? That can't be right."

Others aren't really that surprised. Maybe you haven't been feeling "quite normal" for the past couple of years. Or you were told your blood sugar was high a couple of years ago, and you simply never came back.

And now you feel as if your life has changed—and you aren't quite ready for that. You're concerned about what this will mean for you on a daily basis. How will it affect your job, your family, your relationships, your life? What do you do? What *should* you do?

The diagnosis of type 2 diabetes or prediabetes does change your life—and it should. Although there is a genetic component, these are mainly diseases of lifestyle—which means by making changes to your lifestyle you have the power to determine how things go from here. And if you take this "wake-up call" seriously and make improvements in the way you live, you can extend the years—and the quality—of your life.

There are a lot of books out there that promise that you can "cure" diabetes. I need to tell you up front there is no "cure" for diabetes. By the time you are diagnosed, your body, particularly those cells that are responsible for the regulation of your blood sugar, have been significantly damaged. Yet, with the right lifestyle changes, you may be able to reverse the high blood sugar. You may even be able to avoid prescription medication. Once you're told you have prediabetes or diabetes, however, you'll always need to be vigilant.

I'm not promoting gimmicks or fad diets, as some books do, or asking you to buy expensive equipment with the promise that you will reverse diabetes. Rather, I will provide you with useful tools to develop a strategy that can have a big impact on your overall health. You have the power! What you need is the practical information to use that power properly and take control of your risk. You're about to learn much that you didn't know about prediabetes and diabetes. Some facts might surprise you and others will reinforce what you already know. Get ready to become better informed in new and compelling ways!

You have a diagnosis. You've heard the wake-up call. What's next? What exactly do you need to eat? How much exercise is necessary and what type? Do sleep and stress really affect your blood sugar? Why are you feeling sad? Is this a condition you will have for the rest of your life? The next nine chapters tell you what you need to do.

Let's get started.

CHAPTER ONE

What Exactly Are Diabetes and Prediabetes?

TRUE OR FALSE?

1. Diabetes is the second leading cause of death in the United States.
2. Prediabetes affects more than 100 million Americans.
3. Type 2 diabetes is partly genetic.
4. Type 2 diabetes is uncommon in people younger than twenty-five years of age.
5. Obesity is a major cause of prediabetes.

(Answers at end of chapter)

YOU'RE NOT ALONE. Diabetes and prediabetes are quite common. More than 34 million Americans have diabetes—that's nearly one out of every ten people (see Figure 1). In fact, more than 50 percent of our population has some type of diabetes or prediabetes, and more than 1.5 million people are diagnosed every single year. And the numbers are going up. As a nation and as individuals, we need to get our blood sugar under control. Sadly, we are headed in the wrong direction.

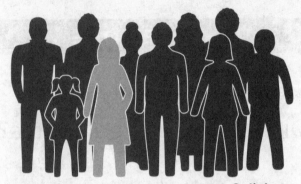

About one in ten people have type 2 diabetes

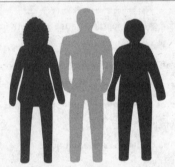

About one in three people have prediabetes

• Centers for Disease Control and Prevention
• National Diabetes Statistics Report, 2020
• Atlanta, GA: Centers for Disease Control and Prevention, U.S. Dept of Health and Human Services; 2020

Figure 1

What's particularly concerning is the number of people who don't yet know they are affected. Of those who have diabetes, more than 20 percent are undiagnosed. Of the 88 million adults with prediabetes, a whopping 84 percent aren't aware their blood sugar isn't normal.

Undiagnosed: Of the 34.2 million adults with diabetes, 26.8 million were diagnosed, and 7.3 million were undiagnosed.

New cases: 1.5 million Americans are diagnosed with diabetes every year.

Nearly 1.6 million Americans have type 1 diabetes:

- 7.5 percent of non-Hispanic whites
- 9.2 percent of Asian Americans
- 12.5 percent of Hispanics
- 11.7 percent of non-Hispanic blacks
- 14.7 percent of American Indians/Alaskan Natives

What exactly is diabetes? And what do we mean by prediabetes?

Despite how common diabetes is, many people don't really understand what's happening in their body. Diabetes relates to how well your body controls blood sugar. I always tell people that diabetes isn't complicated. You need to understand only two things—glucose and insulin. Once you know how these work together, you will have what you need to help manage or even reverse elevated blood sugar.

How do you feel when you haven't eaten in a while? Tired. That's because your cells need energy. Our bodies need energy to survive, and we get that energy primarily from glucose in food. When you eat or drink something, your body breaks down the carbohydrates into glucose, which is then absorbed into your bloodstream.

Your pancreas produces the hormone insulin to help your cells absorb glucose, so that they can use it as energy. Insulin also stores any excess glucose that you don't use right away, mostly in your liver and muscle cells.

The right amounts of insulin and glucose are critical. The two perform a delicate balancing act that requires your body to calibrate the amount of each with expert precision. Too much or too little of either is bad.

We used to think there were only two types of diabetes, but we have now identified at least five types!

1. We have learned over the last few years that type 1 diabetes is an autoimmune disease in which your body attacks and destroys the islet cells of your pancreas, which are responsible for producing insulin. We also know that those who develop type 1 diabetes are genetically predisposed, and that lifestyle plays no role in its development. Type 1 diabetes can develop at any age, but it typically occurs in children and is diagnosed less commonly after one's early thirties.

2. In type 2 diabetes, your body still produces insulin but, because your body has become resistant, it has lost its effectiveness (see Figure 2). To compensate, your body produces more insulin. Even though the insulin amount may be high, it's actually not enough for the amount of glucose you have consumed as well as the amount your body is making, because of your cells' resistance to it. Your liver also produces more glucose, since your cells are not able to utilize glucose effectively. Type 2 represents more than 90 percent of all cases of diabetes.

    Early in my training, I only saw type 2 diabetes being diagnosed in adults. In fact, we used to call it Adult Onset Diabetes. In recent years, however, it has become more common in teenagers. Genetics do play a role but not as much as most people think. Our genes don't change much over decades—it takes generations.

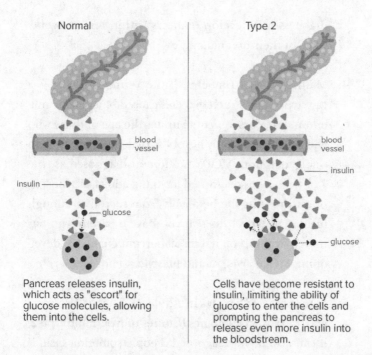

Figure 2

Unlike type 1 diabetes, lifestyle plays a significant role in this type of diabetes. The rise in type 2 cases in young people is directly related to lifestyle—with obesity playing the biggest role. We even created a new word—"diabesity"—to express the relationship between obesity and diabetes.

3. Nearly one in twenty pregnant women develops Gestational Diabetes, likely the result of a combination of factors: less insulin is produced, weight gain makes the insulin that *is* produced less effective, and various other placental hormones reduce the ability of insulin to do its job. Fifty percent of women with gestational

diabetes will develop diabetes within ten to twenty years of their pregnancy.

4. **Maturity Onset Diabetes of the Young (MODY)** is a rare type of inherited diabetes caused by a genetic mutation. It occurs in people under the age of thirty who typically have a family history of diabetes in more than one generation. MODY is often misdiagnosed as type 1 or type 2: it is diagnosed in young adults, as type 2 is, but it prevents the beta cells from secreting enough insulin, as type 1 does. If you have a parent who has this condition, you have a 50 percent chance of developing MODY. Weight and lifestyle do not play a role.

5. **Latent Onset Diabetes in Adults (LADA)** is also rare, and, because it combines features of type 1 and type 2, it can also be misdiagnosed. People sometimes call it Type One and a Half Diabetes! As in type 1, your pancreas stops producing insulin, probably due to auto-antibodies, but it doesn't stop all of a sudden at an early age. Rather, as in type 2, insulin gradually becomes less effective, often resulting in a diagnosis after age thirty. People diagnosed with LADA will often suffer other autoimmune conditions such as ulcerative colitis, Crohn's disease, multiple sclerosis, or rheumatoid arthritis. Your doctor may be able to check by looking for certain antibodies and measuring C-peptide.

Some diseases, such as pancreatic cancer and hemochromatosis, also destroy the cells of the pancreas and cause diabetes— sometimes referred to as secondary diabetes. Others, such as pheochromocytoma, disrupt the way you release insulin.

Cushing's disease and acromegaly can also present with elevated blood sugar. Testing for and treating the underlying disease will likely resolve the episodes of elevated blood sugar.

Some chronic medication use can also cause diabetes, sometimes by causing weight gain, and other times by directly impairing the pancreas. These include glucocorticoids, which reduce insulin sensitivity and cause the liver to produce more glucose, statins, and some antipsychotic and high blood pressure medications.

Finally, there's prediabetes. This is a condition of elevated blood sugar that is likely to become type 2 diabetes if changes aren't made. Nearly everyone who has type 2 diabetes has had prediabetes, although they may not have realized it. One of the goals of this book is to help prevent you from progressing to diabetes if you've been told you have this condition.

Just a reminder: In this book, we are talking about prediabetes and type 2 diabetes. Even though some of the guidance discussed will be helpful for your overall health, the recommendations don't specifically apply to other types of diabetes.

Are You At Risk?

Prediabetes and type 2 diabetes do not occur randomly. Rather, certain factors and behaviors increase your risk. Some you can't control—age, race, and family history—but most you can. Your weight, and high blood pressure or high cholesterol, can increase your risk. Being inactive plays a big role. If you suffer from depression, that can increase your risk. If you have heart disease, you are more likely to develop diabetes, and if you have diabetes, you are more likely to develop heart disease. The good news is that if you reduce your risk of one, you reduce your risk of both.

Several online risk calculators can help you calculate your risk. It's a good idea to take a test to see the impact of different factors. The Centers for Disease Control and Prevention (CDC) and the American Diabetes Association (ADA) have one of the best:

https://www.diabetes.org/risk-test
https://www.cdc.gov/prediabetes/takethetest/

Risk Factors for Diabetes:

- Overweight
- Forty-five years or older
- Parent, brother, or sister with type 2 diabetes
- Physically active less than three times a week
- High blood pressure
- Dyslipidemia (high triglycerides and low HDL)
- Gestational diabetes or have given birth to a baby who weighed more than nine pounds
- Polycystic ovarian syndrome
- African American, Hispanic/Latino American, American Indian, or Alaska Native (some Pacific Islanders and Asian Americans are also at higher risk)

Recent research shows if you are diagnosed with ADHD, you are 50 percent more likely to develop diabetes. It's not clear if the correlation works the other way, meaning if you have diabetes, you are at greater risk of ADHD. This is an emerging area of research, and more study is needed.

In men, stuttering may be tied to early onset of type 2 diabetes. In a study of Israeli youth being evaluated for military service, researchers found a 30 percent greater risk for developing diabetes in men who stutter. No association was seen in women. We aren't sure why risk seems to be increased, but it could be related to stress and cortisol secretion or even changes in dopamine regulation in people who stutter.

Symptoms

What are the symptoms that you should look for? Many people have symptoms for years but don't realize they could be signs of diabetes. By recognizing the symptoms, you can get care sooner, and have a much better chance of preventing or maybe even reversing any progression of diabetes. Here's an easy way to remember the major symptoms of diabetes—they're all "polys":

- Polyuria
- Polydipsia
- Polyphagia

Basically, these words mean you urinate a lot (polyuria), you are often thirsty (polydipsia), and you seem to be more hungry than usual (polyphagia). What's a lot? Most people urinate eight to ten times a day; if you are urinating twelve or more times a day, it's time to get checked. If you seem to be thirsty all the time, even after you drink, your blood sugar may be high. I will always remember my patient Mary, who knew something was wrong. "Dr. Whyte, I was drinking water constantly—and I don't even like water. When I drank from the sink one day, I knew I had to come in!" And if you are constantly hungry, even after you eat—that is not normal, and you need to get checked out.

An important point about weight: although most people with prediabetes and diabetes are overweight or obese, not everyone is overweight. Early on in some people with untreated and undiagnosed diabetes, lack of adequate insulin prevents the body's cells from absorbing glucose in the blood to use as energy. Instead, the body burns fat and muscle for energy, causing a loss in body weight. Your body also dumps a lot of sugar in the urine, reducing your number of calories.

I tell you this because I don't want you to think that if you are not overweight, you can't develop prediabetes or diabetes . . . because you can. About 90 percent of people with type 2 diabetes and prediabetes are overweight, but there are still millions of people with diabetes at normal weight. Please don't ignore symptoms just because your weight seems "healthy."

Other symptoms include:

- Fatigue
- Erectile dysfunction
- Blurry vision
- Repeat yeast infections
- Hair loss or thinning
- Dark skin patches typically on the neck and underarms (acanthosis nigricans)

Remember, you may not experience symptoms of prediabetes. A subset of patients with diabetes reports no symptoms; others have symptoms that are very minor. So, when you are first diagnosed, you may be quite surprised. That's why screening is important.

Diagnosis

We use different lab tests to diagnose diabetes.

You may have heard about the glycosylated hemoglobin or "HbA1c" test. A lot of people just call it "A1c." This test records your average blood sugar level over ninety days—the life of the red blood cell. The result does not represent the percentage of sugar in your blood, but, rather, how much glucose has bonded to the hemoglobin in your red blood cells.

- Diabetes: 6.5 percent or higher
- Prediabetes: 5.7–6.4 percent
- Normal: less than 5.7 percent

Years ago, we only used this test for patients who had already received a diabetes diagnosis, as a way to monitor how well they managed their blood sugar. That was because some labs calculated blood sugar levels differently. We have made progress over the years, and this is now an established diagnostic test.

Take note, however, that since this measurement is related to red blood cells, if you have diseases that affect those cells, such as sickle cell disease or thalassemia, the measurement may be less accurate. This can also happen if you have underlying liver or kidney disease.

Another option is to take a random blood test, one taken regardless of whether you had fasted. If you have symptoms and a blood sugar level greater than 200 mg/dl, you likely have diabetes. If the result of your random glucose test is abnormal, repeat it another day or consider a different test.

Most of the time, your doctor wants a fasting glucose level. Fasting means you have not eaten anything for at least eight hours. I always suggest that patients schedule the lab in the morning because it's easier to fast overnight than during the day. Don't schedule the test for 3:00 p.m. By noon, you will definitely regret that decision.

Results:

- Less than 100 mg/dL is normal
- 100 to 125 mg/dL indicates prediabetes
- 126 mg/dL or above indicates diabetes

Finally, there's also the oral glucose tolerance test, which used to be considered the gold standard. Typically, you will need to fast for eight hours and then have your blood drawn at your doctor's office. Then you will drink a sugary solution—which is never tasty! Don't be fooled by anyone who tells you it tastes like lemonade, because it doesn't! Two hours later, your blood sugar is checked. In another two hours, your blood glucose level is measured again.

Results at two hours:

- Normal blood glucose level is lower than 140 mg/dL (7.8 mmol/L)
- Prediabetes: between 140 and 199 mg/dL (7.8 and 11 mmol/L)
- Diabetes: 200 mg/dL (11.1 mmol/L)

Doctors didn't use the term *prediabetes* in the past, but it isn't a new condition. We did speak of "impaired glucose tolerance" or "impaired fasting glucose" based on the results of the above tests. We were not as aggressive in treating this, since we still didn't fully understand the impact of chronically elevated blood sugar. Now we know better.

Should You Get Screened?

The American Diabetes Association (ADA) recommends that everyone over the age of forty-five be screened for prediabetes and diabetes. The US Preventive Services Task Force recommends that people who are overweight or obese (BMI >25) should begin at age thirty-five. That might be too late for some people. That's why the ADA recommends that adults who are overweight or who have one or more risk factors should be screened whatever their age.

If your doctor doesn't order a test, make sure to tell them you want it. Today, at-home tests that you administer yourself are available, but the tests done through your doctor's office are more accurate.

Early diagnosis is key!

If you are having symptoms and your blood sugar is normal, that doesn't mean you can keep eating junk food and being a couch potato. You should still make lifestyle changes and consider retesting in six months to a year. Otherwise, if you have no symptoms and your blood sugar is within normal range, get screened every three years.

Summary

Both prediabetes and type 2 diabetes are becoming much more common, and are usually caused by poor eating habits and lack of physical activity. Although prediabetes often has no symptoms, diabetes can have a range of symptoms including excessive thirst, urination, or hunger. Everyone over forty-five should be screened for prediabetes and diabetes, and people who are overweight or have risk factors should be screened earlier. There are several tests to diagnose diabetes and your doctor can determine the best time. Abnormal test results should be confirmed by a second test.

ANSWERS

1. **FALSE.** Diabetes *is* considered a leading cause of death in the United States, but it's usually ranked about seventh.
2. **FALSE.** Prediabetes affects more than 80 million Americans, and diagnoses are increasing. I hope we won't reach 100 million.
3. **TRUE.** Type 2 diabetes does have a genetic risk, but it's estimated that genetics contributes to less than 15 percent of cases.
4. **FALSE.** Although people older than forty-five are the most commonly diagnosed, type 2 diabetes is occurring more frequently in people younger than twenty-five. That wasn't the case twenty years ago.
5. **TRUE.** Obesity is the leading cause of prediabetes.

CHAPTER TWO

The Dangers of High Blood Sugar

> ## TRUE OR FALSE?
>
> 1. Eye damage is often the first complication of diabetes.
> 2. People with diabetes are at increased risk of getting carpal tunnel syndrome.
> 3. High blood sugar can cause hearing loss.
> 4. If you're a woman with diabetes, your risk of a heart attack is tripled.
> 5. Complications from diabetes usually take at least ten years to develop.
>
> *(Answers at end of chapter)*

"MONICA" HAS BEEN STRUGGLING with her weight since she's been a teenager. "Dr. Whyte, I've been fat my whole life and only have had diabetes for a year. Other than a few aches and pains, I don't have any problems. Plenty of people I know are in worse shape than me." Monica is correct in that right now she seems to be doing okay. The problem is that chronically elevated blood sugar has a big impact on your long-term health. While it slowly and silently damages tissues, at some point, the symptoms and complications catch up with you, potentially causing many problems.

Your glucose level is not just a number. That's what some patients tell me when I tell them they have prediabetes or even diabetes. "It's just a number. I feel fine." It's true that it is a number but it's a number that has a lot of meaning and impacts your life. I want you to think about it another way. Elevated blood sugar needs to be a wake-up call to improve your health. There needs to be a sense of urgency to reverse and prevent complications. It shouts for you to take control of your risk.

All too often, patients and sometimes even their doctor dismiss the lab result and say "let's retest in a few months." For most people with or at risk for diabetes, blood sugar steadily creeps up if you don't change anything. It's almost as if you don't want to admit what's happening. I have had many others who say "let's wait a while" and then don't come back the following month, and then months turn into years. Some end up in the emergency room with blood sugar in the 500s!

Others attempt to change their lifestyle but their efforts aren't consistent. Let's be honest—it's hard to change our habits as we get older! People don't take medicines as directed, either because they haven't accepted they have diabetes or they just don't think it's that serious. The end result is always serious health problems. Make no mistake—we need to aggressively treat diabetes and even prediabetes because the effects of chronically high blood sugar are quite harmful, and even deadly. We waste too much time because we either don't know what to do, or we simply take too long to develop a practical strategy. I hope that by reading this book, you are changing that!

Complications of Diabetes

Diabetes can lead to many complications (see Figure 3). They can be quite serious and will impact your life considerably if you develop them. That's why it's so important to take control of your blood sugar and manage your risk.

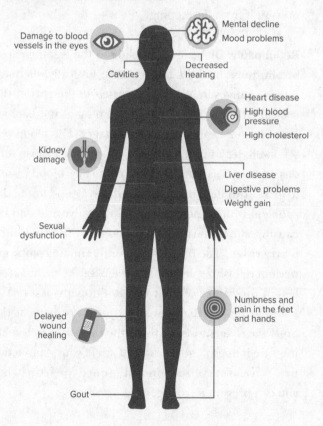

WAYS DIABETES CAN AFFECT THE BODY

Damage to blood vessels in the eyes

Mental decline
Mood problems

Cavities

Decreased hearing

Heart disease
High blood pressure
High cholesterol

Kidney damage

Liver disease
Digestive problems
Weight gain

Sexual dysfunction

Numbness and pain in the feet and hands

Delayed wound healing

Gout

Figure 3

- **Neuropathy.** People with diabetes often report numbness and pain, typically in their feet and hands. It can affect your balance, walking, and writing. The pain often keeps you up at night. This is because high blood sugar damages your nerves. Often it takes years for neuropathy to develop. That's the good news since it allows time to get diagnosed and reverse the high sugar. The bad news is that once you develop diabetic neuropathy, it can be very hard to treat. Medications often treat symptoms but don't reverse the damage. The key is to prevent it from developing.

- **Retinopathy.** Diabetic retinopathy is the leading cause of blindness in the United States. Basically, diabetes causes changes in your blood vessels in the part of the eye called the retina. That's the lining at the back of your eye that changes light into images. The blood vessels swell, leak fluid, or bleed—all of which cause serious damage. Diabetes can even cause new blood vessels to grow. Although this may sound like a good thing, the problem is these new vessels are defective and end up causing more harm. Often people will experience blurry vision, lose the ability to differentiate colors, experience flashing lights, and even suffer from vision loss in the center of their eye. Retinopathy is an early complication of diabetes and is often present at the time one is diagnosed. If that's the case, the key is making sure it doesn't get worse and affect your daily activities. You can't reverse retinopathy once you have it, but you can prevent it from getting worse.

- **Nephropathy.** Our kidneys are essential to staying alive. Damage from diabetes is the leading cause of chronic kidney disease. In the advanced stages of kidney damage, you often either need to undergo dialysis or need a transplant. Nearly a third of people with diabetes also develop kidney disease, so avoiding elevated blood sugar levels is a must. People tend to think that kidney disease affects their ability to urinate, and it does eventually—but it often causes many more problems before you notice that symptom. Some people will develop swelling of their face, as well as hands and feet, because the body isn't controlling fluid balance well. Others might feel tired due to a low blood count, since your kidneys can no longer make enough of the hormone needed to form red blood cells. You often will have nausea and trouble sleeping. It's a good idea to have your urine tested at least yearly for albumin if you have prediabetes or diabetes to keep watch on your kidneys. But there are many other health consequences that often arise much sooner.

- **Weight gain.** As I mentioned earlier, most people who develop prediabetes or type 2 diabetes are overweight or obese. In fact, nearly nine in ten are. It becomes a vicious cycle: extra weight can trigger elevated blood sugar— and that will usually lead you to gain even more weight. In the early progression of the disease, people remark how it makes them hungry. Some patients who are already overweight will occasionally ask me if more weight really matters that much. Yes, it does. Obesity is so common nowadays that many people don't think it's that big a deal, but it is. Numerous studies have shown that a

higher body mass index (BMI) is associated with increased risk of death. Even more compelling is the relationship between mortality and *central* obesity—that's fat
around our midsection. If you can "pinch an inch," your
risk of more complications increases significantly.

- **Heart disease.** This is the most serious complication of
diabetes and the one that many people are familiar
with. We now consider diabetes a risk factor for heart
attack just as we do high cholesterol and high blood
pressure. The risk for a heart attack is more than double for men with diabetes than it is for men without
diabetes and more than triple for women with diabetes.
Over time, high blood glucose from diabetes damages
your blood vessels and the nerves that control your
heart and blood vessels, putting you at risk for a heart
attack. Heart disease is the number one cause of death
in people with type 2 diabetes. Anyone diagnosed with
prediabetes or diabetes should work with their doctor
to determine their heart disease risk, which plays a big
role in how aggressive you need to be treated.

- **High blood pressure.** We are used to thinking that only
sodium contributes to high blood pressure, but sugar is
another culprit. High blood sugar causes our arteries to
stiffen, damaging their lining—that can make your
blood pressure rise. High blood pressure dramatically
increases your risk of strokes and heart attacks.

- **High cholesterol.** Diabetes does the exact opposite to
our body when it comes to our cholesterol goals—it
raises triglycerides and lowers good cholesterol. It also

changes the characteristics of bad cholesterol, making LDL smaller and more dense, which makes it easier to enter the walls of arteries, causing plaque. Part of it may be the food we eat, the weight we gain, and the impact on our arteries and liver. It can also be a result of high blood sugar affecting the enzymes that help break down or make cholesterol. Getting to know your lipid levels is important to help you take control of your risk. Don't become too preoccupied with your lipids if they are normal. It turns out that the HbA1c level I mentioned earlier may be a better predictor of heart disease than your cholesterol and LDL levels.

- **Liver disease.** The kidney isn't the only organ that high blood sugar damages. Persistently high blood sugar is associated with developing nonalcoholic fatty liver disease (NAFLD), a condition that causes swelling and, in advanced stages, scars your liver. We may think of liver disease as a risk among people who drink alcohol but NAFLD, as the name implies, occurs in people who drink little or no alcohol. It's becoming much more common in people with diabetes—nearly half of people with diabetes will develop it. Make sure your doctor measures your liver enzymes since we are starting to see that high liver enzymes increase diabetes risk.

- **Insomnia.** If you are having trouble sleeping, prediabetes or diabetes may be the culprit. Blood sugar spikes and crashes can also make it more difficult to stay awake. Chronically elevated blood sugar also decreases the amount of deep sleep, causing you to be less refreshed when you wake in the morning. It can turn into a vicious cycle, where poor sleep makes it hard to control blood sugar and poor blood sugar control makes it hard to sleep.

- **Cavities.** Too much sugar has long been associated with tooth cavities. The sugar interacts with bacteria in your mouth to create acid that wears away tooth enamel. It's not just cavities, though, that you need to be concerned about. Diabetes also weakens gum muscles, which can result in tooth loss. We now know that oral health is associated with overall health and cavities can be a sign of other health conditions.

- **Carpal tunnel syndrome.** Within the last few years, we have seen an increased incidence of carpal tunnel syndrome and some other orthopedic issues, such as tendon rupture, in people with diabetes. This most likely is a result of nerve damage. If you are diagnosed with prediabetes and you develop carpal tunnel syndrome or rupture a tendon, your likelihood of progressing to diabetes is increased.

- **Mood problems.** The relationship between blood sugar and mood has been well established. How do you feel right after you've eaten sweets, and how do you feel a few hours later? It's not just about the short-term effects of high blood sugar but also the long-term effects that we need to worry about. Several studies have shown that people who consume more than the equivalent of twelve teaspoons of sugar daily are nearly 25 percent more likely to be diagnosed with anxiety or depression. We aren't exactly sure why this occurs, but we do know that too much sugar can cause swelling and inflammation in the area of the brain associated with mood. We also know that a diagnosis of diabetes, or even pre-diabetes, can make you depressed so it works both ways.

- **Gout.** I bet you associate gout with the "good life"—consumption of red meat, wine, lobster. Mmmm . . . yum! But it's also associated with high blood sugar, especially if you are insulin resistant. People with type 2 diabetes often have high levels of uric acid in their blood. That extra uric acid can form crystals in your big toe, wrist, knee, and other joints. Gout flares can cause significant pain and disability. Experts estimate that women with gout are 71 percent more likely to get diabetes than women without it.

- **Kidney stones.** As with gout, chemicals in your urine are responsible for kidney stones. Those chemicals develop solid crystals, which cause writhing pain in the back and groin. Studies show that having type 2 diabetes more than doubles your chances of developing certain types of kidney stones. Possible reasons include a more acidic urine as well as insulin resistance in people with diabetes. Believe me—you want to avoid getting kidney stones.

- **Delayed wound healing.** Many people seem to know someone with diabetes who has lost a limb. Typically, a patient develops a small ulcer or wound, and then several weeks later, the affected limb has to be amputated. Diabetes impairs circulation, preventing oxygen and other nutrients from reaching wounds, and that causes slow healing. Cells can't access enough glucose and that can lead to infection as well. Amputations are more common than you think: more than two hundred patients with diabetes undergo amputation each day!

- **Gastroparesis.** This is a big word but simply represents a condition in which your digestion slows down and food stays in your body longer than it should. It occurs because the nerves that move food through the digestive tract are damaged, so muscles don't work properly. As a result, food sits in the stomach undigested. This often results in heartburn, nausea, and vomiting. Guess what the most common cause is? Diabetes.

- **Cancer.** In recent years, researchers have noted a relationship between diabetes and some types of cancer (for example, pancreas, endometrium, colon and rectum, breast, bladder, and non-Hodgkin's lymphoma). Although it's overly simplistic to say cancer cells need sugar to survive, insulin resistance and inflammation due to obesity and high blood sugar likely play a role in developing some cancers.

- **Parkinson's disease.** New data suggests that people with diabetes are at increased risk of developing Parkinson's. It can be as much as 32 percent more likely. What's even more concerning is that type 2 diabetes may be associated with faster progression, due to the risk of a more aggressive form. There's some belief that insulin might help protect your brain, and if you have insulin resistance, you aren't as protected. Abnormal protein function can also play a role.

- **Decreased hearing.** High blood sugar can cause damage to the nerves in the ear, resulting in difficulty hearing. Keep in mind that hearing impairment is associated with early dementia—so the more we can do to keep our hearing intact, the less chance of developing dementia.

- **Sexual dysfunction.** High blood sugar can make it more difficult to get or maintain erections. This is likely due to damage to nerves and small blood vessels. Men with diabetes typically develop erectile dysfunction issues ten to fifteen years earlier than men without diabetes. For women, prediabetes and diabetes can damage the nerves that create sexual excitement and stimulation. The good news for both men and women is that if you get your blood sugar under better control, you can often reverse this and regain sexual function.

- **Vaginal itching and infections.** Elevated blood sugar often causes vaginal dryness and itching. This is likely a result of sugar in the urine, which can be a breeding ground for yeast infections. When women complain of frequent vaginal infections, checking glucose levels is typically a good idea.

- **Decreased skin quality.** When you have chronically elevated blood sugar, you don't produce enough keratin. Skin may feel thin, rough, dull, and dry. Your body may also lose its ability to control how much melanin you produce, making certain areas darker. You also lose some subcutaneous fat, especially around your shins.

- **Aging.** Diabetes causes you to age? Yep, that seems to be the case. People who consume a lot of sugar—perhaps by drinking lots of soda, eating candy, and snacking on cookies—have shorter telomeres. Telomeres are caps at the end of our DNA that help to protect our cells. Most telomeres get shorter over time, during the natural process of aging. High-sugary foods, lack of physical activity, and chronic inflammation tend to shorten the length of your telomeres and that can shorten your life.

- **Osteoporosis.** Diabetes changes the mineral composition of bones and reduces new bone formation and bone strength, and increases risk of bone fractures. Postmenopausal women are particularly susceptible. Osteoporosis occurs more often in patients with type 1 diabetes but we also see it in people with type 2.

- **Hair thinning.** There are many reasons why one might develop hair loss or thinning of the hair. In diabetes, your follicles don't grow and reproduce as quickly, resulting in a weakened texture. Your immune system can also start attacking hair follicles, resulting in receding hairlines.

- **Mental decline.** A growing body of research shows an association between prediabetes and mental decline occurring earlier than it does in people who don't have prediabetes. Prediabetes can also increase your risk of vascular dementia, which is caused by reduced blood flow to the brain. Prediabetes is not associated with increased risk of Alzheimer's disease but diabetes is. Patients with type 2 diabetes are more likely to have a decrease in certain areas of the brain that are linked to Alzheimer's. The most recent data suggests that the risk for dementia increases considerably if diabetes is diagnosed at a younger age, particularly if you do not control your blood sugar well. This is likely due to the longer duration of poor glucose control. Having poorly managed diabetes for more than ten years can double your dementia risk by the time you are seventy.

One other point to keep in mind is that if you have diabetes and you are hospitalized, your risk of dying is increased. This increased mortality doesn't even depend on the reasons for admission.

I don't tell you about these conditions to scare you but to fully inform you. If you act quickly and stay focused, you may likely avoid many, if not all, of these complications. If you ignore high blood sugar and don't work hard to reduce it, you could be decreasing your quality of life. Studies have shown that if you have an HbA1c greater than 7 percent and don't do anything to reduce it, at five years, your risk of a stroke, as well as a heart attack and heart failure, increases dramatically. That's why I want you to act and reduce risk! Find out how in the next few chapters.

Summary

Diabetes can result in serious health conditions, including damage to your heart, brain, liver, eyes, kidney, skin, stomach, and hair. You may have begun to experience some health issues by the time you are diagnosed, or within a few years of diagnosis. The longer your diabetes is poorly managed, the greater your risk of damage to your body.

ANSWERS

1. **TRUE.** By the time people are diagnosed with diabetes, many already have signs of eye damage.

2. **TRUE.** People with diabetes are at increased risk of getting carpal tunnel syndrome.

3. **TRUE.** High blood sugar damages nerves through the body, including in the ear, which can cause hearing loss.

4. **TRUE.** Diabetes significantly raises your risk of a heart attack, especially if you are a woman.

5. **FALSE.** Most people with diabetes start to develop some complications within just a few years of their diagnosis.

CHAPTER THREE

The Truth About Cure and Reversal

TRUE OR FALSE?

1. Type 2 diabetes is lifelong. Once you have it, it's here to stay.
2. Once you have prediabetes, developing type 2 diabetes is unavoidable.
3. You can cure yourself of diabetes.
4. Nearly everyone with diabetes develops complications.
5. Every year, about 10 percent of people with prediabetes reverse it and return to normal blood sugar.

(Answers at end of chapter)

BETTY IS FIFTY YEARS OLD and about fifty pounds overweight. Other than some knee pain, Betty has developed few symptoms, and to her credit, she has done pretty well with her health. But four years ago, her blood sugar as well as HbA1c were elevated, putting her in the prediabetes category. "Tell me what to do, Doc, and I will do it." Over several months, Betty and I discussed ways to change what and how much she eats. We also discussed the different types of exercise she needed to perform and their frequency. At first, Betty was seeing improvement in her blood sugar control. But around six months later, Betty's blood sugar started to increase again. "Ugh, this is hard work. I'm not sure what I'm doing wrong." Betty was adamant she didn't want to start medication. "Once I start, I will never come off, will I?" she would ask.

After some coaxing, Betty decided to take her lifestyle changes up a notch. She talked to a nutritionist to help with meal planning and signed up for some online exercise classes. Within a couple of months, she lost ten pounds and her blood sugar was improving. Roughly a year and a half after being told she had prediabetes, her blood sugar returned to normal, and has remained normal for the past year. When I asked her about this success, she remarked, "To be honest, I wasn't sure I could do it, but I kept at it. I needed to get rid of this diagnosis."

But did Betty "get rid of" her diagnosis?

A lot of books and online sites promise a "cure" if you follow some special diet, or a reversal without taking any medications. "Just make a few simple changes and you can prevent complications and reverse the effects of high blood sugar." Seems too good to be true, right? Well, the short answer is *it depends*.

Before we talk about potential reversal or cure, I need to explain what happens to your body before you are diagnosed since a lot is going on before symptoms develop or you get an abnormal lab test.

Due to a combination of your personal risk factors including age, genetics, weight, and lifestyle, your body slowly stops processing glucose correctly. One major culprit: the beta cells in your pancreas, which are responsible for making insulin, start to go haywire.

Because your body isn't responding to glucose well, the beta cells start pumping out more insulin to get your body to use the glucose. It's like when your cell phone starts to lose its charge—you keep trying to charge it more by leaving it plugged in more often. Early on this works, and your blood sugar remains normal but at the expense of excess work by your pancreas. At some point, though, this strategy stops working and you no longer can compensate by putting out more insulin.

Your beta cells become impaired—they either get burned out, die, stop functioning properly, or morph into another type of cell (see Figure 4). Now, you can't secrete as much insulin to keep up with the demands required to help keep your sugar normal. Your body is still not responding to insulin, which means your cells can't utilize glucose well and your liver releases more glucose to help. Simply put, you no longer make enough, and your body doesn't respond effectively to the

PROGRESSIVE LOSS OF BETA-CELL FUNCTION OVER TIME

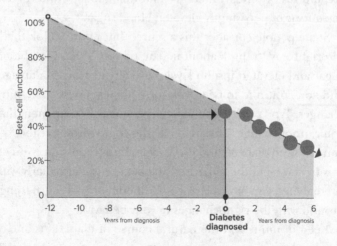

Figure 4

insulin you *do* make. A double whammy! All that insulin has other effects that come into play that make diabetes a condition that is more than just about your blood sugar.

By the time type 2 diabetes is diagnosed, your body has been having problems with glucose and insulin for at least five to ten years. Most patients' beta cells will have lost about 40 to 50 percent of their function and, without adequate intervention, will continue to lose another 5 percent per year. The end result: worsening blood sugar levels and the beginning of damage from diabetes. This is one of the reasons why screening for diabetes and diagnosing prediabetes is so important. Stop the course of diabetes early on and you change the outcome. You have the power to avoid permanent damage to the cells.

Here's some good news: blood sugar in prediabetes and diabetes can be reversed to normal under certain circumstances!

We used to think that once beta cells burned out and lost function, that was the end of them. If that's the case, we would never be able to reverse or prevent the complications. But we now have evidence that these critical cells may indeed regenerate and restore their function—and that allows you to reverse the effects of persistently elevated blood sugar.

Some people consider this a "cure," but I don't think that's the right way to think about it. The reason is that high blood sugar and elevated insulin levels have already caused damage, and you continue to be at risk for diabetes unless something changes. Type 2 diabetes also has a genetic risk component that you cannot change. I like to make the comparison to cancer— you can send diabetes and prediabetes into "remission." You do this by reversing the impact on the beta cells. Particularly with prediabetes, you have a chance—a limited one—to turn things around with the right changes in your behavior.

Keep in mind that the natural course of diabetes is one of progression—and not in a good way. As discussed in chapter 2, diabetes can affect nearly every part of your body. When the damage occurs varies. Some people have complications at the time of diagnosis, some develop them within five years, and still others may avoid complications for twenty years. It depends on many factors, so try not to compare yourself to others. I've noticed over the years that everyone seems to think they will be the one that doesn't develop complications for many years, or if they do, they will be minor. Perhaps you also think "It won't be me." The reality is that most people develop complications within five to ten years of diagnosis. (Remember, the problems with the pancreatic beta cells start much sooner than diagnosis.) Sadly, the result is often a shortened life and/or decreased quality of life.

But if you take active steps to change the course, you may be able to reverse prediabetes and/or diabetes or prevent or delay complications. I'm more encouraged about potential reversal than I was ten years ago. And that's because we have lots of research that shows when certain action is taken and sustained—especially early on—it's possible for many people to reverse course.

Consider the National Diabetes Prevention Program (National DPP) for insights about reversing prediabetes. The researchers with the National DPP attempted to evaluate how intensive lifestyle changes compare to medication in preventing the progression of prediabetes to diabetes. With more than twenty-five research sites around the country and thousands of participants, this study served as a landmark trial that changed how we think about reversal! They split participants into three groups—the control group received no specific intervention; the second group received the drug metformin; and the third received intensive lifestyle coaching that included a low-calorie, low-fat diet and at least 150 minutes per week of moderate-intensity exercise.

The goal of the lifestyle group was to lose 7 percent of their baseline body weight. The results were impressive! Forty to fifty percent of them were able to return to a state of normal glucose regulation that lasted for several years, and for some, decades. The lifestyle group did the best of all three groups—it even out-performed the group that received medication to lower blood glucose levels. What I find particularly encouraging is that those who were able to reverse their prediabetes and normalize their glucose regulation showed a 56 percent lower risk of developing type 2 diabetes than those who maintained blood sugar in the prediabetes range. In people over sixty, lifestyle changes resulted in a 71 percent reduction in diabetes risk! Even after ten years, the risk reduction was 34 percent. Again, just 7 percent weight loss. For someone 175 pounds, that's roughly 12 pounds.

A more recent study teaching lifestyle changes in a group support setting had similar results. It included patient-centered counseling techniques, motivation to change, social support and assistance with goal setting, action planning, and self-monitoring. The goal again was 7 percent weight loss for most people, 150 minutes per week of moderate-intensity exercise including two to three sessions of muscle strengthening, and healthy eating. There were twelve hours of educational group sessions. Most participants were followed for two years. No medications were prescribed.

Again, impressive results in reversing high blood sugar! In fact, there was a 40 to 47 percent reduction in the risk of developing type 2 diabetes in those who participated in the study.

I want you to see that these and other studies have shown that the more you are able to return to normal glucose regulation, the greater the likelihood you can prevent type 2 diabetes.

Let's be realistic—you might not get it right the first time. Sadly, people often give up when they don't immediately get the results they hoped for. But numerous studies show that achieving normal glucose levels dramatically reduces your risk of progressing to type 2 diabetes. Please don't get discouraged if you don't succeed the first couple of times you try. No one suggests this is going to be easy. The chapters in the book are designed to give you the tools to help. But it does take time. Keep at it and the benefits will follow.

The key is to act now—don't wait. You bought this book and now you need to implement what's in it. Most experts agree that the best window of opportunity to prevent or slow the progression of prediabetes to type 2 diabetes is about three to six years after you've been diagnosed. Doing nothing will likely lead to full-blown diabetes. In general, about 10 percent of people with prediabetes progress to diabetes each year, and according to an ADA expert panel, up to 70 percent of individuals with prediabetes will eventually develop diabetes if they don't manage it. In a diabetes prevention trial conducted in China, the twenty-year cumulative incidence of diabetes was even higher, greater than 90 percent.

Fortunately, the same strategies for reversing prediabetes can also be used to put type 2 diabetes into remission. The Diabetes Remission Clinical Trial (DiRECT) evaluated patients in the United Kingdom with type 2 diabetes diagnosed for less than six years and who were not taking insulin. This study found that nearly 50 percent of the participants who underwent a structured weight-loss program led by their primary care physician were able to achieve remission of their diabetes after one year. In this case, remission was defined as an HbA1c less than 6.5 percent and off all diabetic medications for at least two months. The researchers also found that the more weight lost, the greater the chance of achieving remission. For example, 34 percent of participants who lost 5 to 10 kg (approximately 11 to 22 pounds) of body weight achieved remission while 86 percent of those who lost 15 kg (around 33 pounds) or more achieved remission.

What's particularly exciting about this trial is that further analysis of DiRECT showed that beta-cell function can return to normal in response to weight loss. Researchers used MRI images to evaluate pancreas volume and fat content, both of which improved significantly with weight loss. Insulin secretion also improved, a necessary step for reversal. Other studies found that in patients with type 2 diabetes who lost considerable weight and achieved remission, their beta-cell function matched that of non-diabetic subjects.

The Look AHEAD trial (Action for Health in Diabetes) also evaluated the effects of lifestyle changes involving diet and exercise on diabetes control. In this study, lifestyle intervention was compared to diabetes support and education. The group of subjects who underwent lifestyle intervention scored significantly better on weight loss, physical fitness, and body fat mass metrics than those who only received support and education. These changes translated into improved quality of life and less intense medication management in diabetic patients. At one year, remission was 11 percent.

So how can beta-cell function be assessed? Some studies suggest that the proinsulin:insulin ratio is one way. Measuring C-peptide levels in the blood is another way. It's best to talk to your doctor about what tests are most appropriate for you.

Weight-Loss Surgery

Some people, despite their best efforts, won't be able to lose weight and keep it off to achieve remission of prediabetes or diabetes. Some people will be candidates for bariatric surgery, often referred to as weight-loss surgery (see sidebar below). Most procedures involve either rerouting your digestive tract to bypass the stomach or reducing the size of the stomach. Because your stomach is smaller, you cannot eat as much, and you feel "fuller" sooner. Some procedures are reversible and some are not—so you need to consider this option very carefully. As it relates to diabetes, improvements in blood glucose are often seen just days after the surgery is performed, even before significant weight loss. Some experts believe it may be related to the changes in hormones released in your stomach and intestines.

As many as 70 percent of bariatric surgical patients go into diabetes remission within six months and often maintain normal glucose and insulin levels for at least five years. People who have had diabetes for less than three years and who aren't taking insulin before surgery seem to do best. Bariatric surgery is considered major surgery, and does have some risks, both short and long term. For example, people can develop vitamin and mineral deficiencies. Keep in mind it is not a treatment for prediabetes.

INDICATIONS FOR BARIATRIC SURGERY

- BMI ≥ 40, or more than one hundred pounds overweight.
- BMI ≥ 35 and at least one or more obesity-related comorbidities such as type 2 diabetes, hypertension, sleep apnea and other respiratory disorders, nonalcoholic fatty liver disease, osteoarthritis, lipid abnormalities, gastrointestinal disorders, or heart disease.

I don't want you to think that it's only about weight loss, and that once you get to a healthy weight, diabetes automatically goes away. Remember, prediabetes and diabetes relate to how your body responds to insulin. Weight is a major factor but not the only one.

Role of Medications

In recent years doctors have been more frequently prescribing medication early, after a diagnosis of prediabetes, given that many people cannot make or sustain lifestyle changes, and the risk of developing diabetes is high. I tell patients the key is how can we help you return to normal blood sugar—that's what is critical. Ideally, we can do it with the lifestyle changes we are discussing in this book. If so, that's great. But if you can't make healthy lifestyles changes to the degree necessary to return to normal insulin and glucose levels, we can't just let prediabetes turn into diabetes. In that circumstance, you need to speak with your doctor about the role of medication.

Even with lifestyle changes, some people will need medication to manage their type 2 diabetes. Medications can play an important role for many people, even as they make lifestyle changes. Don't think that it's either medications or lifestyle. It depends on a variety of factors and your personal medical history. Having worked at the US Food and Drug Administration for many years, I can assure you that we continue to develop safe and effective drugs to help manage diabetes and its complications. Some of these drugs can also help you lose weight and decrease your risk of heart disease. Whether you take them is a decision you should make carefully with your doctor. Please don't fear medications or resist taking them if your doctor prescribes them. The use of specific medications for managing diabetes is beyond the scope of this book.

Two Big Don'ts

Prediabetes and diabetes are caused by many factors, including genetic predisposition and hormone regulation. Don't blame yourself and don't let anyone blame you. It's the combination of many things including your genes and your environment that also determine whether you get prediabetes or diabetes. That's why you may know some people who seem to eat bad food all the time and seem fine. (Granted, you don't really know their overall health, but that's a different story.)

Focus on *your* health and not on what other people seem to be doing. Since you can't change your genes, you need to change your lifestyle. That's how you empower yourself. That's what we are doing together to help you take control of your risk.

If you are told your blood sugar is high, please don't ignore it. I have known many patients over the years who don't believe their diagnosis, don't want to admit it, and don't do anything about it. Prediabetes and diabetes are progressive—and I don't mean that in a nice way! They get worse over time and don't disappear on their own. But with the right information, a positive mindset, and some smart approaches to healthy living, you can likely avoid complications—and possibly even turn things around.

Summary

You have the power to reverse prediabetes and even diabetes. It typically requires around 7 percent weight loss, along with several lifestyle changes. The key is to make these changes early on to prevent progression. Some people will need medication in addition to lifestyle changes. Ignoring high blood sugar puts you at significant risk for complications. Even if you are able to return to normal blood sugar, once you've been diagnosed, you will need to remain aware of your lifestyle choices and continue to engage in behaviors that maximize your health.

ANSWERS

1. **FALSE.** Type 2 diabetes can be put into remission by making some effective lifestyle changes and losing excess weight. It's possible to lower your HbA1c below the range for type 2 diabetes and reduce or completely eliminate the use of diabetic medications. You don't need to struggle with diabetes for life, but these changes need to be part of a lifelong strategy.

2. **FALSE.** Prediabetes can be reversed to a state of normal glucose regulation. Being diagnosed with prediabetes does not mean that you are destined to have diabetes! Lifestyle changes, including diet and exercise, can promote this reversal, sometimes with the help of medications. Think of prediabetes as a warning stage; there's still time to take action!

3. **FALSE.** A cure doesn't truly exist. Type 2 diabetes has a genetic component, so you still need to be vigilant and manage it after you have been diagnosed or after you go into remission.

4. **TRUE.** Although the time frame varies, nearly everyone with diabetes develops some complications. The longer you have uncontrolled blood sugar, the more serious the complications you likely will develop.

5. **TRUE.** About 10 percent of people with prediabetes return to normal blood sugar control every year.

CHAPTER FOUR

Your Daily Food Choices Determine Your Future

TRUE OR FALSE?

1. Eating too much sugar causes diabetes.
2. Artificial sweeteners often help people lose weight.
3. The ketogenic diet is the best diet to control high blood sugar.
4. Intermittent fasting can help reduce your risk for diabetes.
5. Coffee can increase your risk of diabetes.

(Answers at end of chapter)

FOOD IS MEDICINE.

Food is medicine.

Food is medicine.

If there is only one concept from this book that you must remember, it's this: everything you put into your mouth can affect your body in either a good or a bad way. The food you eat helps determine how your brain functions, how fast your heart beats, how strong your muscles and bones become, how well your liver and kidneys get rid of toxins, and even whether your pancreas produces too much or too little insulin.

Don't quite believe me, or think I'm exaggerating? How do you feel after eating a bunch of candy? I bet the resulting sugar rush feels pretty good. But then an hour or so later you crash.

Do you need coffee in the morning to help start your day? What happens if you miss that morning brew? I bet you drag throughout the day and may even get a headache. And who doesn't get sleepy after Thanksgiving dinner?

Yes, what you put in your mouth affects your whole body.

You can't take control of your risk for prediabetes and diabetes if you don't manage your daily food choices. And to be honest, it's not just the impact on diabetes that's important. There is a wealth of data showing the effect of your food choices on heart disease, cancer, brain disease, and mental health.

Food can be as powerful as prescription drugs.

Given the importance of a healthy diet in reducing your diabetes risk or reversing prediabetes, I must tell you up front that this is not the book that is going to tell you that you can eat whatever you want. I know there are some diet books out there—and even some doctors—that lead you to believe that, but it's simply not true. If you want to keep your blood sugar within normal range, watching what you eat plays a critically important role. Your food choices can protect your health, and they can also harm your health. I want to give you the information you need to choose foods that maximize your health and reduce risk of disease. Remember, persistently elevated blood sugar leads to diabetic complications. So, let's use every strategy to get your blood sugar to stay at a normal level.

"Tell Me What to Eat."

FOODS TO INCLUDE

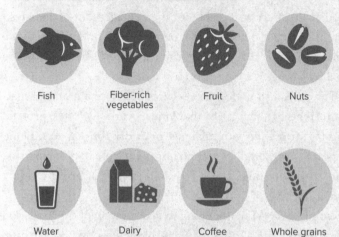

Fish

Fiber-rich vegetables

Fruit

Nuts

Water

Dairy

Coffee

Whole grains

FOODS TO CUT BACK ON

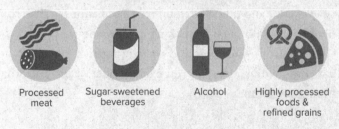

Processed meat

Sugar-sweetened beverages

Alcohol

Highly processed foods & refined grains

I hear that a lot from patients. I always think of that old Italian proverb: "teach him how to fish and you feed him for a lifetime." I'm not trying to be flippant, but for you to be successful—to take control of your prediabetes and diabetes risk—you need to learn how to create a diet for yourself that meets *your* needs.

Recognizing the need for personalization, the American Diabetes Association (ADA) published a consensus report in 2019 that reviewed the scientific evidence behind different diets and their impact on diabetes and prediabetes. Their conclusion: "A variety of eating patterns (combinations of different foods or food groups) are acceptable for the management of diabetes." There's no diet that will work best for everyone but there are *general principles* that are important to follow when it comes to healthy eating.

The ADA also no longer specifies a precise amount of macronutrients to aim for—by that I mean, carbohydrates, protein, and fat for people with diabetes, or at risk for diabetes. Limiting carbohydrates does play an important role in reducing risk, but "carb counting" is not required as part of healthy eating principles.

Don't worry—I'm not going to take away all of the foods you enjoy and create a category of "forbidden foods." But, realistically, you are going to need to make some changes—and for many of you, they may be big changes. That may be a shock at first, but think about it—would you rather take a pill or injection every day and potentially suffer complications or take control of your blood sugar by making healthy choices?

When it comes to food and preventing risk, it's all about what you include and what you exclude. Let's start with what you should include.

Fish

One of the best dietary changes you can make to help control your risk of developing diabetes is to eat fish. Less than 20 percent of Americans eat eight ounces of fish weekly. Fish is full of vitamins, omega-3 fatty acids, and minerals like potassium, zinc, and magnesium. It's also low in calories, which is good for your waistline. I tell patients if you replaced one serving of meat a week with a serving of fish, you'd be well on your way to weight loss and better blood glucose control.

Patients often ask me what kind of fish. There are so many options nowadays. Some of us didn't grow up eating fish so we aren't quite sure of what our choices are. Others express concern about contaminants. Ahi tuna, tilefish, king mackerel, and swordfish tend to have higher levels of mercury than other fish, so you want to limit consumption of these particular fish, but the levels of contaminants in most varieties of fish, either farmed or wild-caught, are too small to cause harm. Salmon, flounder, tilapia, trout, and even sardines can be part of your diabetes prevention program. You can even use tuna or salmon in a can or pouch for convenience. The benefits of eating fish, however, are going to outweigh any risks, especially if you eat it in moderation. You should try to have at least two servings of fish per week—again, *replacing* red meat, not as surf and turf!

Sometimes people are unsure of how to cook fish. There are plenty of options: grilling, baking, broiling, sautéing, poaching, even microwaving. Just don't deep-fry them. Fish sticks are not going to count toward your healthy eating plan either!

Fiber-Rich Vegetables

How many vegetables did you eat today? I bet the answer is less than two. Ideally, you should aim to eat at least three servings of vegetables a day—but the more the better. (It's weird math but, technically, one-half cup of cooked vegetables or one cup of raw vegetables counts as one serving.) Non-starchy vegetables like broccoli, carrots, leafy greens, brussels sprouts, peas, cabbage, cauliflower, asparagus, and mushrooms are some of your best options because they're chock full of fiber, vitamins, and minerals, and they have a minimal impact on blood sugar levels. One of the reasons why I encourage fiber-rich vegetables is that they slow the rate at which your body absorbs sugar from food, preventing potentially harmful spikes in blood sugar after meals. Studies have found that if you have diabetes or prediabetes, you can lower your risk of an early death by consuming plenty of dietary fiber. In a recent review of studies, researchers looked at data on almost a million people and found that those who consumed the highest levels of fiber had a 23 percent lower mortality rate than people who consumed the least. Each 10-gram increase in fiber intake was associated with an 11 percent lower risk of dying early.

Fruits

For some reason, a lot of people with prediabetes or diabetes have been told that they need to be careful about eating fruit. Please don't fear fruit! The truth is that you *can* and should eat fruit. Several recent studies have demonstrated that daily consumption of fruit decreases the risk of diabetes by 5 to 12 percent. And for those who have diabetes, eating fruit three days per week has been shown to reduce complications by 28 percent. Pretty impressive, isn't it? Yet, only 10 percent of Americans get even two cups of fruit every day. When did you last have an orange or a banana? I know I struggle many days, and often need to make an effort to eat a piece of fruit. I've learned to get into a habit of having some fruit in the morning.

Fruit—especially whole fruit—has so many benefits. Just as with certain vegetables, the fiber minimizes the effects of natural sugar. Fruit has flavonoids, which are powerful antioxidants that fight off toxins that cause damage to our cells and blood vessels, and is rich in essential nutrients like vitamins A, C, and E, as well as folate, zinc, magnesium, and potassium. At the same time, fruit is low in fat, and low in calories. I can go on and on. I think you can see why fruit is so important when we talk about controlling your diabetes risk.

Some of my favorite choices that offer the most bang for the buck are those with a dark color—blue, purple, and red: blueberries, blackberries, plums, and cherries.

And in case you are wondering, tomatoes count as a fruit *and* a vegetable. Double benefit. ☺

Go ahead and eat fruit! Honestly, I don't get too worried about someone eating too much fruit. It's always going to be a better choice than eating potato chips and candy bars. Fruit is Mother Nature's candy. One piece of advice: avoid fruit juices (and yes, that includes the ones labeled "100 percent juice"). Juice processing removes a lot of the fiber as well as some nutrients. As a result, the sugar is absorbed more rapidly in your cells and can lead to spikes in your blood sugar.

Nuts

Nuts are a healthy snack. I don't mean to disappoint you, but chocolate-covered almonds or salted cashews are not what I'm talking about. Nuts are a great source of protein, fiber, and healthy fats. Some nuts, such as almonds and pistachios, even contain melatonin (which promotes healthy sleep cycles). Other nut varieties contain vitamin E, magnesium, and potassium. Patients often tell me they don't eat nuts because nuts contain a lot of fat and a lot of calories—and that is true. But moderation is key. What's moderation? Typically, a handful is a healthy amount. Some data has shown that people with diabetes who eat nuts five times a week reduce their risk of heart disease, probably by reducing inflammation and oxidative stress. Just remember—peanuts are not nuts, they are legumes, which are plants that produce a pod with seeds inside.

Water

Did you realize your body is more than 50 percent water? That makes your daily water consumption quite important. If you're like me, you need to drink more water. The US National Academies of Sciences, Engineering, and Medicine determined that an adequate daily fluid intake is about 15.5 cups (3.7 liters) of fluids a day for men. And about 11.5 cups (2.7 liters) of fluids a day for women. Are you thinking what I'm thinking? That seems rather high! For most people, drinking eight 8-ounce glasses a day (about 2 liters or 1/2 gallon), should be sufficient, especially since you consume some water through food.

Why is water important to reduce your diabetes risk? There are a couple of reasons. Water has no sugar and zero calories, which will help prevent weight gain. When you drink enough water, it can dilute the amount of sugar in your blood and help eliminate excess glucose through your urine. This all helps to get your blood sugar under control and prevent spikes.

You have lots of choices nowadays when it comes to drinking water. Flavored, sparkling, tap—it's all good as long as there is no added sugar. You may remember a few years ago when people were promoting coconut water to prevent diabetes or at least keep blood sugar low. We haven't had any scientific studies to support these claims, so I don't recommend coconut water, especially since some varieties contain a bunch of sugar. Keep it simple—regular water is all you need.

Dairy

We know that dairy is good for our bones, since it is a rich source of calcium and vitamin D. Now we know it might also help you reduce your diabetes risk. Consuming dairy—particularly yogurt—can help you manage diabetes and even prevent development of prediabetes. A large study of the diet habits of health professionals followed over many years seems to indicate that a diet rich in dairy may protect you from developing type 2 diabetes. The researchers found that consuming dairy seems to be especially beneficial if it is consumed during your teen years and early adulthood. Don't worry, though, if you haven't been eating Greek yogurt lately! You can still benefit from dairy even in your fifties and sixties. Here's a tip someone gave me a few years back: try incorporating string cheese or cottage cheese into your diet. Also, go ahead and drink that milk, preferably skim or 2 percent. Just as long as it's not chocolate milk!

Coffee

All you coffee drinkers, take note: we have strong evidence that drinking coffee lowers the risk of type 2 diabetes.

Drinking one to two cups of coffee each day may lower the risk of developing type 2 diabetes by 4 to 10 percent. This is likely due to the antioxidant and anti-inflammatory effect of coffee. It also helps your body release more insulin and respond better to the insulin you do release. As a result, it decreases your body's resistance to insulin, which is one of the factors in developing diabetes. Most data shows benefits, as long as you don't drink more than two to three cups a day. If caffeine makes you jittery, you can still can get some benefit with decaf, although not as much. Remember, mocha cappuccinos and double-shot

vanilla lattes do not count! For those of you who don't like coffee or want to try something different, I've got a good option—
tea! More than two-thirds of the world's population drink tea.
Tea contains polyphenols, which are also powerful antioxidants.
Several studies have shown that drinking three to four cups of
tea a day can reduce one's risk for diabetes.

Whole Grains

We tend to eat a lot of grains in the United States. The problem
is we're not eating enough of the *healthy* ones to reduce diabetes risk. That's a mistake, since recent data shows that whole
grains might reduce the risk of diabetes by 22 to 34 percent.

The word *whole* is what makes the critical difference. The
grain is "whole" when it has not been refined or processed.
That's important because whole grains have much more fiber
and vitamins than processed or refined grains. They help your
cells respond more effectively to insulin. Since fiber is hard to
break down, it also makes you feel full sooner, stopping you
from overeating. Ideally, you should get 25 to 30 grams of fiber
a day, and at least half should be from whole grains.

When you spend some thinking about it, why would we
choose anything other than whole, since the process of refining
removes all the good stuff!

How do you know which are the whole grains? It's actually
kind of simple. Look for products labeled "whole grain" (don't
be misled by labels that say "multigrain" or "12 grain"—look
specifically for "whole" to get the most benefit).

That's what you should include. Not too complicated, is it?

You might be thinking, "I don't like fish" or "I tried nuts and
they weren't for me." "Milk upsets my stomach." I've even had
a patient tell me she didn't like water. Guess what? Taste is

acquired. Although some anthropologists may disagree with me, you're not pre-programmed to like potato chips and despise peas. A few years ago, I was trying to switch from whole milk to skim milk. When I first tried skim, I thought it tasted like water. It wasn't until I drank it and used it in my cereal every day for about two weeks that my taste buds adjusted, and I began to prefer skim. When I then tried whole milk again, I was like, "Yuck. This tastes like I'm drinking cream." Just as our kids often need to try a food seven to ten times to know whether they like it, we need to do the same, and not dismiss these healthy food options after one or two tries.

Some pundits out there like to promote the idea of sugar as an addiction. The reality is that sugar is not addictive: our bodies do not become physiologically dependent upon it. Sugary treats can be hard to resist, and many people find it quite tasty. But sugar is not addictive. Calling it such diminishes the active role you can play in directly choosing the right foods to help reduce your prediabetes and diabetes risk.

These points are important because you've learned to like certain foods, which means you can also learn to unlike them.

What are certain foods you need to unlike?

Here are the foods you need to cut back on to reduce your risk of prediabetes and diabetes.

Processed Meat

Processed meat is one of those foods that you will need to eat less of if you want to decrease your prediabetes and diabetes risk. Research has shown that each 50-gram (1.8-oz) daily serving of processed meat (about one to two slices of deli meats or one hot dog) was associated with nearly a 20 percent higher risk of developing diabetes.

Marketers can fool us with names of products that sound healthy—but no matter how you label bacon or sausage, they're still not good for you. For instance, products often are labeled "nitrates- or nitrites-free"—which makes you assume that the risk is gone. The risk may be reduced, but it's not eliminated since nitrates/nitrites are not the only component that increases risk. Although they don't usually contain sugar, processed meats tend to be high in fat and heavy on salt and preservatives—things that help to give flavor. These have been linked to an increased risk of type 2 diabetes.

Many of us grew up eating lunchmeats on white bread, and some of us still pack those sandwiches for lunch. It seems convenient, doesn't it? But, instead of relying on the prepackaged lunch meat, a better choice would be to go with a fresh, leaner cut of meat and see it sliced off the bone. Try using leftovers from a roasted turkey or grilled chicken breast. Convenience is important, but so, too, is the long-term impact on your health.

You may be wondering about red meat. It has been shown to be associated with heart disease, certain types of cancer, *and* diabetes. Some experts believe it's related to the heme iron in meat, and others think the method of cooking is responsible for the risk. High temperatures involved in barbecuing and roasting may release certain chemicals that decrease your body's sensitivity to insulin. The more red meat you eat per week, the greater your risk. Red meat, however, does contain some important nutrients, particularly protein, and some B vitamins, so occasional consumption is okay. When you do choose red meat, try to select the leanest cuts and eat small portions. According to the USDA, the leanest beef cuts include round steaks and roasts (eye of round, top round, bottom round, round tip), top loin, top sirloin, and chuck shoulder and arm roasts. For ground beef, the label should say at least "90 percent lean."

Sugar-Sweetened Beverages

This one should be pretty obvious, yet many patients with diabetes continue to drink soda, lemonade, fruit juice cocktails, and sweet tea. "They quench my thirst," Patsy likes to tell me. "I'm from the South," Jim remarked to me. "We drink sweet tea all day." We know these beverages can wreak havoc on your blood sugar due to the high carbohydrate content and the high calories. They also provide an easy way to consume 300 to 400 calories in a few gulps without even realizing it.

Can you solve the problem by just switching to the "diet" versions of your favorite beverage? I wish it were that simple, but it isn't. Science has consistently shown that people who drink diet soda often still gain weight. Some studies have even shown that participants who started out at a normal weight and drank three diet sodas a day were *twice as likely* to be overweight or obese years later as their non-diet-soda-drinking peers. That seems counterintuitive, doesn't it?

Data suggests that people overestimate their calorie savings from choosing diet beverages. How many of us have ordered a double cheeseburger and fries, and then said "diet coke" as if that somehow magically negates all those calories? I'm sorry to tell you it just doesn't work that way—I wish it did but alas, it doesn't!

What About Artificial Sweeteners?

Artificial sweeteners are much sweeter than sugar. Some are two hundred times as sweet, and others are up to ten thousand times as sweet. You read that correctly—ten thousand times! That taste tricks your brain to tell your pancreas to release insulin—and since you don't actually have any glucose around, the insulin can make you crave sugary treats. If you've been wondering why you want a cupcake with that diet soda in the afternoon, that might be why!

My goal for you is not to switch to diet drinks, but to water. Here's a strategy that might help wean you off diet beverages and replace any type of sweetened beverages with water—it worked for me a couple years go: try flavored water (adding lemon or lime) or sparkling water. There are plenty of fruit-infused waters on the market—you will likely find one you'll enjoy. Just make sure you choose one with no added sugar. Honestly, it will take some time to get used to the switch—possibly two to three weeks—but you can and should do it. Our desire for sugary drinks is learned—we aren't programmed at birth to want them. This also means we can unlearn these preferences!

Alcohol

You may be aware of the connection between alcohol and liver disease, but you may not be aware of the link with diabetes. While some amount of alcohol can make your blood sugar rise, especially since some beer and wine (and particularly cocktails!) contain carbohydrates, too much alcohol over time can cause low blood sugar, especially if you have diabetes. Although alcohol can decrease the effectiveness of insulin, excessive alcohol consumption makes it harder for the liver to produce glucose; combine that with the decreased food consumption that sometimes goes hand in hand with heavy alcohol use, and you now have a situation where blood sugar can get too low.

I'm not suggesting you can't drink alcohol, but you should stay within the moderate range. Moderate alcohol consumption is defined as no more than one drink a day for women and two drinks for men, no more than five days a week. One drink is defined as one 12-ounce beer, 5-ounce wine, or 1.5-ounce distilled spirit.

Highly Processed Foods and Refined Grains

This is probably not a surprise: prepackaged, processed foods are typically high in fat, salt, and sugar. This may help them taste better, but eating too many of these foods may increase your risk of prediabetes and complications from diabetes. They often contain unhealthy additives such as hydrogenated oils, modified starches, colorants, and texturizers. Reducing intake of processed foods, especially those ultra-processed ones, will improve your overall health. As for refined grains, I'm not a fan. Remember—refining takes out all the good stuff—fiber, vitamins, and minerals. Examples of refined grains include many breads, crackers, baked goods, and white rice. If you are like most people, processed and refined foods compose more than half of the foods you eat. It should make you think twice about eating too much processed food and refined grains.

That's what you need to cut back on eating if you want to cut back on your risk for prediabetes as well as diabetic complications.

I don't want you to read this and think you can never eat a hot dog or a few cookies, or that by eating a steak and drinking a glass of wine, you're going to get diabetes. That's not the case. Rather, it's your consistent daily choices, over time, that make the impact. If you eat bacon for breakfast most days, and drink three glasses of wine every day, and drink soda at lunch, you are increasing your risk of diabetes. Remember: food is medicine! What you put in your mouth is going to impact your body in ways that may takes years to show. You likely won't feel the effects of your food choices for some time. That can make it hard to associate what you eat now with your health later.

Supplements—"Food in a Pill?"

A lot of dietary supplements advertise that they can help you prevent diabetes or better manage the disease. I hate to be the bearer of bad news, but most of those supplements do not have evidence behind them. And for the few that do, the evidence is mostly weak. Let's take a quick look at what works and what doesn't work, starting with those that might provide some benefit.

One of the most popular supplements that is marketed for diabetes is chromium. An essential mineral found in many foods, chromium helps your body metabolize carbs and fats and regulate blood sugar levels. Dozens of clinical trials have examined its potential benefits. In a recent analysis, researchers reviewed all the data and found that taking 200 micrograms of chromium daily could slightly improve glucose levels in people with poor blood sugar control. It also lowered triglycerides and raised HDL (good) cholesterol. The scientists did not find much evidence of serious side effects. But they warned that more research looking into the long-term safety of taking chromium supplements was needed.

Another supplement that has been found to offer minor benefits for diabetes is alpha lipoic acid, a substance found in meat and some leafy green vegetables. Studies have found that taking alpha lipoic acid can help with diabetic neuropathy and potentially improve insulin sensitivity. It's not exactly clear why. But it may have something to do with its ability to reduce the accumulation of triglycerides in skeletal muscle, which is one of the underlying causes of insulin resistance. While alpha lipoic acid is generally considered safe, it can cause gastrointestinal distress if taken in large doses. So keep that in mind.

Now let's look at some supplements that don't live up to the hype. If you have diabetes or prediabetes, then you've probably heard that cinnamon (which, yes, is technically a spice) can lower your blood sugar levels. There's been plenty of research looking into this claim and, unfortunately, it just isn't borne out. In a recent well-designed study, researchers recruited seventy adults with type 2 diabetes and randomly assigned them to one of two groups. One group was instructed to swallow cinnamon capsules daily, which amounted to them ingesting about 1 gram of cinnamon each day. The other group was given a placebo. After sixty days of this, the researchers found that the cinnamon didn't have any impact at all on HbA1c or fasting blood sugar levels. So how should you interpret this data? First off, don't go and toss any bottles of cinnamon out of your spice cabinet just yet. It's a wonderful spice that is chock full of taste. You should still use cinnamon if you already like it, especially as a replacement for salt or sugar. Just don't waste your money on cinnamon supplements, and don't expect that dumping tons of it on your food will do anything to improve your blood sugar control.

There's a long list of other supplements that miss the mark: bitter melon, fenugreek, ginseng, milk thistle, and various Chinese herbal medicines. The National Institutes of Health has concluded that studies haven't proven any of these supplements to be effective, and some may have side effects.

What about omega-3 supplements, sometimes referred to as fish oil supplements? Over the years, the data relating to heart and brain health and diabetes has been mixed. In a recent review of more than eighty randomized trials involving more than one hundred thousand people, the use of omega-3 supplements did not show an impact on the development of diabetes. This is still an evolving area of research so more information may be available in a few years, but what does seem clear is that the pill form of omega-3 doesn't offer the same benefit as the natural version found in foods. This is an important point for people who don't want to try fish—you can't get the same benefits from a pill. Just doesn't happen.

Unfortunately, the story is much the same for many other popular supplements that have at times been promoted for other conditions and now are being suggested for diabetes treatment and prevention. At least eight different trials have found that vitamin D had no impact on glycemic outcomes in people with diabetes. And a meta-analysis of fourteen clinical trials found that vitamin E did not significantly improve HbA1c, blood sugar, or insulin levels. I could go on, but I think that by now you get the picture. What you eat determines your risk of diabetes and how your body handles the disease. But when it comes to supplements, there is no magic pill.

Microbiome

What about our guts? Everyone seems to be talking about the microbiome. What role does it play in managing your diabetes risk?

The trillions of microbes that live in and around our bodies, collectively known as the microbiome, play a critical role in our overall health. The largest concentration of these microbes resides in the gut, where they have a direct impact on blood sugar levels, inflammation, body fat, and insulin sensitivity. Some of these microbes live in harmony with us. They produce compounds that benefit us and in return we feed and house them. But others are like unwelcome squatters who spew toxins into the bloodstream, wreaking havoc on your metabolism and helping to set the stage for diabetes.

I mentioned earlier that systemic inflammation is a component of risk for diabetes, which can be influenced by what happens in the gut. The microbes that live in the gut may be our inhabitants, but they are technically not part of us: they are different species with their own DNA. When they remain safely in the gut, they can provide a lot of benefits. But if they slip past the gut's protective barrier and enter the bloodstream, it becomes a different story. When that happens, the immune system treats them as foreign invaders and launches a series of inflammatory processes—the same steps it would take to vanquish any other potentially dangerous germs.

What keeps this from happening is the lining of your gut, a thin mucosal membrane known as the epithelium. This barrier is made up of cells that are lined up side by side with tight junctions between them, allowing nutrients to pass through while at the same time keeping microbes safely contained in the gut. Studies show that people with type 2 diabetes often have leaky, damaged gut barriers, which drives inflammation throughout the body. One reason is that diabetics tend to have lower levels of beneficial microbes that protect the lining of the gut. The names of these microbes can be a mouthful, but they are worth knowing. Three of them are *Bacteroides vulgatus*, *Bacteroides dorei*, and *Akkermansia muciniphila*. Together these bacteria help to keep the junctions in the lining of the colon tight, which reduces its permeability. Meanwhile, two other species, *Faecalibacterium* and *Roseburia*, produce a compound called butyrate that is critical for metabolic and digestive health. Butyrate helps to keep the integrity of your gut lining intact. It also promotes hormones that stabilize blood sugar levels. Studies show that people with diabetes tend to have very low numbers of these important microbes.

Even when they remain inside the gut, these microbes can play a direct role in the inflammation that is typically seen in diabetes. Some particularly nasty strains of microbes in the gut produce compounds known as lipopolysaccharides, or endo-toxins, which get absorbed into the bloodstream, causing an inflammatory response from the immune system. But other microbes have a much more beneficial effect. Some stimulate the production of interleukin 10 (IL-10), a compound that has powerful anti-inflammatory properties. They also suppress in-flammatory molecules like C-reactive protein and Tumor Ne-crosis Factor alpha. And they influence blood sugar levels. *Akkermansia*, for example, helps prevent the breakdown of com-plex carbohydrates, which keeps blood sugar from spiking after meals. Other important bugs, which people with diabetes tend to lack, produce enzymes and hormones that improve insulin resistance and glucose tolerance.

By this point, I know what you're wondering. How can you transform your microbiome into one that will help you stave off diabetes? Unfortunately, there is no magic bullet: it's not clear from studies that popping probiotic supplements can cultivate a healthy and enviable microbiome, and a recent systematic review of clinical trials raised questions about the safety and effectiveness of probiotic supplements. The one safe and proven method that we know is to eat a healthy diet. We know from high quality studies that following a nutrient-dense diet with plenty of fiber and whole foods will populate your gut with microbes that enhance your metabolic health. Your gut bugs love fiber. It's their favorite source of food. When they get plenty of fiber, they use it to churn out beneficial compounds like butyrate, the compound I mentioned earlier that protects against cancer and diabetes. But when your gut bugs don't get enough fiber, they go into starvation mode and chew on the lining of your intestines. That results in a leaky gut and systemic inflammation. To avoid that, focus on a high-fiber diet that will keep your gut microbes happy and healthy—vegetables, beans, nuts and seeds, as well as lean meats, seafood, and fermented foods we've been discussing. Eating such fermented foods as plain yogurt, kefir, kimchi, tempeh, miso, and Gouda cheese is a great way to support your microbiome because they contain live cultures, which seed your gut with healthy microbes. Studies show, for example, that people who regularly eat plain, unsweetened yogurt have higher levels of beneficial bugs. Beans, nuts, and leafy greens will increase some of the other friendly gut bugs that I mentioned. So, from now on, whenever you're getting ready to eat a meal, remember that you are not just feeding yourself, but the trillions of microbes that live in your gut. Choose wisely!

I mentioned at the beginning of the chapter that the ADA doesn't recommend any specific diet for people with diabetes or prediabetes. Rather, the key is to follow guidelines, like those I just reviewed. Yet, over the years, I still get questions about whether you should try a specific diet. At least every few months, someone asks me, "Should I try keto? My friend did and she lost fifteen pounds."

What about keto?

Ketogenic Diet

The ketogenic diet, or "keto" as some people call it, has become one of the trendiest diets around. It's immensely popular in fitness circles and a buzzword among health and wellness influencers on social media. Keto is often touted as a quick way to lose a lot of weight, but it's also notable for the striking impact that it has on blood sugar levels. That's because it's essentially an extreme form of low-carb dieting that requires slashing your carb intake, typically all the way down to 5 percent of your daily calories, or the equivalent of about 50 grams of carbs, the amount in a single cup of rice or pasta. It's also high in fat. In the case of keto, the diet lowers blood sugar levels so much that it pushes your body to produce ketones, a form of energy that your cells can use in addition to glucose. For people with diabetes and prediabetes, the impact can be dramatic—at least in the short term.

In one meta-analysis of dozens of studies, scientists found that people assigned to follow low-carb diets (defined as restricting carbs to less than 40 percent of daily calories) had greater declines in HbA1c compared to people assigned to follow higher-carb diets. They also had greater improvements in their triglyceride and HDL cholesterol levels and were also more likely to reduce their diabetes medications. The effects on HbA1c were most striking during the first year of a low-carb diet, but over time, the effects on HbA1c petered out, and the difference in HbA1c between the low-carb and higher-carb groups largely disappeared. It is not clear why. It could be that it gets harder and harder for people to avoid carbs in a world that is awash in carb-rich foods, or the weight loss that people initially experienced has been regained with the consumption of non-carb calories. I want you to adopt a style of healthy eating for a lifetime, and I don't think keto works for most people with prediabetes or diabetes. Healthy eating should not be that hard or restrictive. Not to mention the bad breath that sometimes comes with ketones!

After reading about the need for fruits and vegetables, you might be thinking the same thing at least a few patients a year ask me: "Would I be healthier if I became a vegetarian?"

Vegan & Vegetarian Diets

I bet you have thought about going "vegetarian" at some point in your life. I think we all do. Vegetarian is a word that can encompass a range of eating styles. Vegans will not eat any foods derived from animals—some don't even eat honey, because it is made by bees. Vegetarians on the other hand eat mostly plants but will typically make exceptions for things like cheese, milk, and eggs. Then there are people who eat mostly plant foods but occasionally will consume fish. Regardless of which one of these approaches you follow, there is good evidence that cutting back on meat and filling your plate with plants can help to reduce or prevent diabetes. One of the reasons, according to studies, is that plant-based diets typically lead to weight loss.

Meta-analyses of long-term trials have found that vegan and vegetarian diets help people shed pounds while also reducing their waist circumferences, HbA1c, and bad cholesterol levels. In one study, researchers recruited seventy-four adults with type 2 diabetes and assigned them to follow either a calorie-restricted vegetarian diet or a conventional low-calorie diet. After six months, they found that people on the vegetarian diet lost more weight and had greater improvements in their insulin sensitivity. They also had greater reductions in both surface-level and internal body fat. Perhaps most striking, 43 percent of people on the vegetarian diet reduced their need for diabetes medication, compared to just 5 percent of people on the control diet. If you have diabetes or are at high risk for the disease, then following some variation of a plant-based diet will likely benefit your health.

Now you have a good sense of what you should and should not be eating. But does timing matter? Should you be fasting as everyone seems to be doing nowadays?

Intermittent Fasting

Although fasting has been in vogue for the past few years, people have been fasting for religious reasons for thousands of years. Now it's also a popular thing to do for health reasons, in part because a growing number of studies show that it can help you lose weight, improve your cholesterol, and lower your risk of developing diabetes. Should you give a try? Here's what you should know.

The first thing to know about intermittent fasting is that there are several different ways to do it. One popular approach is the 5:2 diet, which involves eating normally for five days a week and fasting for two. Another version of the diet, alternate-day fasting, entails eating less than 500 calories every other day. There's also a regimen called time-restricted eating. People who follow this approach, often called TRE, eat within a relatively narrow window of time every day, typically no more than eight hours, followed by a sixteen-hour fast. Any form of fasting will in theory lead to weight loss because you'll end up eating less food. But some experts claim that there are additional benefits that go beyond the reduction in caloric intake.

At least two large studies involving overweight women compared the 5:2 diet to a traditional low-calorie diet. In both studies, the women lost similar amounts of weight on each diet over a period of six months. But the studies also showed that women who followed the 5:2 diet had greater reductions in their waist sizes and more substantial improvements in their insulin sensitivity. In other words, the authors concluded, the 5:2 diet is at least as good as a standard low-calorie diet for reducing your risk of diabetes. In another study of the 5:2 diet, researchers recruited adults with type 2 diabetes and assigned them to either fast for two days each week or consume no more than 1,200 to 1,500 calories daily. After a year of this, the researchers found that people were just as likely to lose weight and lower their blood sugar levels on either diet. In fact, both groups had similar amounts of weight loss and improvements in their HbA1c, suggesting that the diets were roughly equivalent for diabetes management.

Alternate-day fasting is also quite popular, and studies show that it might offer some benefits. But of all the types of intermittent fasting, it may be the most difficult one to follow. In one of the largest and most rigorous clinical trials of this form of fasting, researchers recruited one hundred obese adults and assigned them to one of three groups. One group was instructed to reduce their daily caloric intake by about 25 percent. The other was assigned an alternate-day fasting regimen in which they were to consume just 25 percent of their daily caloric needs on "fasting days" and allowed to consume up to 125 percent of their caloric needs on "feast days." The third group, which served as the control, did not follow a new diet: they were told to maintain their weight and their eating or exercise habits throughout the trial. The results were rather interesting. After a year, nearly 40 percent of the people in the alternate-day fasting group dropped out of the study—compared to just 29 percent of people in the low-calorie group and 26 percent in the control group. For many people, the alternate-day fasting regimen was no walk in the park. The researchers did see improvements in those who stuck with the fasting program through the entire study, but it wasn't easy to do. But they also were comparable to the outcomes in the low-calorie group: Both diets led to similar improvements in body weight, insulin resistance, blood pressure, heart rate, triglycerides, inflammation, and blood sugar and insulin levels. But the fasting group had significantly higher levels of LDL cholesterol, something that may require further study.

Finally, there is time-restricted eating. It doesn't require that you go entire days without eating much food. You can still consume three square meals and even snacks. But you do have to consume all your food in a limited window of time, typically about eight hours, which generally leads people to consume fewer calories overall. Studies have shown that this form of fasting tends to have a beneficial effect on appetite and satiety, in part because it reduces levels of ghrelin, the so-called hunger hormone. But there is a catch. It seems that to benefit from this diet you will have to implement what's known as an "early" eating window, one that involves eating for example from 8 a.m. to 2 p.m., rather than from 2 p.m. to 10 p.m. The reason for this is that eating earlier in the day aligns with your circadian rhythm, which primes your body to respond better to food in the morning and afternoon rather than at night. Your body increases its production of insulin in the morning, for example, and then gradually reduces its release of insulin in the evening. A number of other hormones and enzymes that are important for metabolism follow this daily pattern as well. That's why it is better to consume most of your food earlier in the day, when your body is prepared to metabolize it.

Like everything else, fasting has drawbacks as well as benefits. Because it necessitates going extended periods of time without eating food, it may cause some muscle loss—which would be bad for anyone, but especially someone who has diabetes or prediabetes. So, if you do try intermittent fasting, you should prioritize eating protein during your "feast" periods to help minimize any potential muscle loss. And lastly, if you use insulin to control your diabetes, then definitely don't try any form of intermittent fasting unless you've discussed it with your doctor: it could lead to serious medical complications.

Food Labels

When's the last time you looked at a food label?

If it's been more than a few months, I hope I can change that. If you want to reduce your risk of prediabetes and diabetes, you need to start looking at them. You don't need to be spending a lot of time on them—rather, here's a quick way to do it that also allows you to compare food choices.

First, look at the number of calories. The important point here is that you need to look at amount per serving as well as the number of servings per container. It will require some math but if it's 250 calories per serving and there are three servings—that's a whopping 750 calories.

Does this mean you need to count calories? I don't typically advise this—or do it myself—since I feel that's not how most people think about food. Rather I do try to have an awareness of roughly how many calories I eat a day. When it comes to weight loss—an important component of controlling your prediabetes risk, as well as diabetic complications—you need to create a calorie deficit. Although both exercise and healthy eating are important, most weight gain is driven by the amount of food you eat. Unless you control what you eat and decrease your number of calories consumed, you aren't going to lose significant weight and keep it off.

In general, women typically consume 2,000 calories a day, and men 2,500 calories. That number may vary slightly based on various factors such as your age and activity level. There are about 3,500 calories in a pound. If you want to lose a pound a week, you need to reduce your food consumption by 500 calories a day or burn off that amount with exercise. Eating fewer calories often results in weight loss more quickly.

The next thing is to look at total carbohydrates. Although "carb counting" isn't required anymore, you should still have a sense of how many carbs you are consuming at each meal. Scanning the food label can help. For most people, 300 grams of carbohydrates is the maximum amount you should consume in a day. For people with prediabetes or diabetes, try to get that number much lower, perhaps around 200 to 225 grams.

You may notice that dietary fiber is included under total carbs. I usually subtract that amount since fiber isn't digestible so it doesn't raise your blood sugar. A good goal for fiber is around 30 grams per day.

Pay careful attention to the total sugars and added sugar section.

According to the FDA, added sugars include sugars that are added during the processing of foods (such as sucrose or dextrose), foods packaged as sweeteners (such as table sugar), sugars from syrups and honey, and sugars from concentrated fruit or vegetable juices. (The FDA also points out that it doesn't include naturally occurring sugars that are found in fruit, vegetables, and milk.) Bottom line: it's usually added calories without added nutrients. You want to keep the amount very low—ideally below 25 grams a day.

Be wary of "sugar-free" labels. Of course "sugar free" can be a healthy choice, but such products can still contain calories and carbs. The key is to confirm what else it contains and then make your decision.

Finally, look at ingredients and see if you can pronounce the words. You may not have realized that food manufacturers are required to list them by amount, from most to least. Be sure you recognize the ingredients as real food.

One of the best uses of food labels is to compare products. For instance, if one type of yogurt has 25 grams of carbs per serving and the other has 10 grams, the choice should be obvious.

---

8 FOODS THAT SOUND LIKE HEALTHY CHOICES BUT OFTEN ARE NOT

- **Bagel.** It's basically a donut. Lots of refined carbs and too many calories.
- **Veggie sticks.** Unlike real vegetables, they have little fiber and too much salt. Protein is low too.
- **California sushi roll.** No healthy fats in this roll and way too many carbs.
- **Beef jerky.** The extra protein is counterbalanced by excessive sodium.
- **Yogurt-covered raisins.** These contain quite a sugar load. Consider it candy.
- **Rice cakes.** They're low in calories and also low in nutrients.
- **Spinach wraps.** Very little spinach and very little fiber. The green is mostly from food coloring.
- **Granola bar.** The healthy nuts and oats are often combined with artificial ingredients and excess sugar to help bind it all together.

Plant-Based Burgers

Have you tried one of those Impossible Burgers or Beyond Meat options? More and more people are trying these plant-based alternatives. But can you kill two birds—eat burgers *and* consume healthy nutrients—at the same time, and even decrease your risk for diabetes and prediabetes? The answer is "maybe." Here's why: the National Institutes of Health found the imitation meats to be a better source of fiber, folate, and iron than ground beef. But imitation meats also have less protein, zinc, and vitamin B_{12}—and lots of salt and saturated fat. They also contain many more carbs than real meat. They are also highly processed to provide the color, texture, and flavor of meat. It's a matter of personal taste, but you probably can't count these as part of your healthy eating plan.

Food Logs

Occasionally I ask people to keep a food log. At first, folks are very resistant to the idea. "I don't have time for that!" is the usual response accompanied by a rolling of eyes. But keeping a food log, or food diary, in which you record everything you eat for a week, can play an important role in reducing your prediabetes risk and more effectively managing your diabetes. Several apps are available to help you so that you don't even have to write everything down. Some allow you to simply take a picture. The reason I like food logs is they show you how much you eat. After patients itemize their daily eating habits, they often tell me, "I didn't realize I ate that much." I use their logs to look at the following:

- How much fruit did you eat daily? Did you eat it at breakfast? Lunch? Dinner?
- How many trips to fast-food restaurants did you make over the week?
- Did you drink soda and how much?
- Did you eat chips or candy more than three days of the week?
- How many cups of water did you drink each day?
- How many times did you eat fish for lunch or dinner? How many times did you eat meat for lunch or dinner?
- Did you consume any nuts or beans?
- How much bread did you eat each day?
- How many times did you eat after 8:00 p.m.?
- Did you consume any ice cream?
- What vegetables did you eat for breakfast, lunch, and dinner?

There's no judgment and you don't need to impress anyone. A log gives you a quick assessment of how much and exactly what you are eating, and that information can then help you make improvements.

Planning

Eating healthily does take planning. And it takes time to make shopping lists and buy the right foods. I usually try to plan out the week on Sunday. Sometimes I do it on Saturday. I've learned over the years that I need to have healthy foods in the house if I want to eat healthily. Try to decide ahead of time what you will eat for lunch and dinner so you don't need to ask "what should I eat?" a few minutes beforehand, and then make unhealthy choices. Fast food and unhealthy choices often win when you are in a rush. Planning is time well spent as you take control of your diabetes risk. The next chapter will give you some ideas, and even includes what you need to buy to create a month of healthy menus.

Summary

Food is medicine. If you want to take control of your diabetes risk, you must make healthy food choices daily. This means more fruits, vegetables, fish, low-fat dairy, nuts, and whole grains. It also means less processed meat, sugar-sweetened beverages, refined grains, and processed foods. Don't waste your money on supplements unless you have a known deficiency. Take a look at food labels and definitely compare products. Make sure you have a plan for what and when you eat.

ANSWERS

1. **FALSE.** Eating too much sugar can lead to obesity, which is a risk factor for both prediabetes and diabetes. But as noted in the first chapter, obesity is not the only risk factor. Several others, including genetics, contribute to your overall risk.
2. **FALSE.** Most data show that artificial sweeteners do not help most people lose weight.
3. **FALSE.** There's no one best diet to control blood sugar.
4. **TRUE.** Intermittent fasting has been shown to help reduce risk for prediabetes, likely due to the weight loss from decreased calories.
5. **FALSE.** Coffee can decrease, not increase, your risk of diabetes.

CHAPTER FIVE

Meal Planning Made Easy

"WHAT CAN I EAT?" I mentioned that's a phrase I often hear from patients. To help answer that question, I have provided a four-week meal plan. I've included healthy options for breakfast, lunch, and dinner as well as snacks. I've made it easy by also including a shopping list as well as recipes, so there is little guesswork.

Some of you might choose to follow it very closely. Others will pick and choose what they like. Both are reasonable approaches. For instance, even though I include different options for breakfast, if you just want to eat oatmeal for breakfast every day—that's a good choice too! I've intentionally added spices and flavors that you might not be familiar with—I hope you give them a try. Some recipes may look daunting at first—but you will find most take typically less than fifteen minutes in prep time.

I have added the nutritional background to help you with your choices. It might be a good idea to compare what I'm suggesting as meal choices versus what you are eating now.

Go ahead and experiment with these different meals. I think your taste buds—and your waistline—will thank you!

Shopping List

Week One

Produce

- [ ] 1 carton fresh blueberries
- [ ] 2 oranges
- [ ] Small bunch of grapes
- [ ] 1 apple
- [ ] ½ cup blackberries or raspberries
- [ ] 2 heads romaine
- [ ] 4 medium onions
- [ ] 1 head of broccoli
- [ ] 2 packages baby carrots
- [ ] 2 cartons cherry tomatoes
- [ ] 3 cucumbers
- [ ] 1 bunch celery
- [ ] 1 zucchini
- [ ] 1 avocado
- [ ] 8 bell peppers
- [ ] 1 carton strawberries
- [ ] 2 bananas
- [ ] 1 peach
- [ ] 1 watermelon
- [ ] 1 tangerine or orange
- [ ] 1 sweet potato
- [ ] 1 pineapple
- [ ] 1 bunch asparagus
- [ ] 1 carton spinach
- [ ] 3 eggplants
- [ ] 1 carton mushrooms
- [ ] Fresh cilantro
- [ ] Fresh basil

Pantry

- [ ] Olive oil
- [ ] Bread flour
- [ ] Baking soda
- [ ] Baking powder
- [ ] 1 sugar-free vanilla instant pudding mix (5 oz. package)
- [ ] Canola oil
- [ ] Unsweetened applesauce

- ❏ Cinnamon sucralose blend
- ❏ 1 package almonds
- ❏ Ground flaxseed
- ❏ Raisins
- ❏ Hummus, your choice flavor
- ❏ White vinegar
- ❏ Light mayo
- ❏ Light bleu cheese dressing
- ❏ Tzatziki sauce
- ❏ 1 pouch or can tuna
- ❏ Fruit cups in water
- ❏ Pretzels
- ❏ Graham crackers
- ❏ Ranch
- ❏ Teriyaki sauce
- ❏ 8 cups spaghetti sauce (low sodium)
- ❏ ½ cup marinara sauce
- ❏ 4 cups Italian-seasoned bread crumbs
- ❏ 1 package croutons
- ❏ 2 cans tomato sauce (8 oz. cans)
- ❏ 2 cans low-sodium red kidney beans (15 oz. cans)
- ❏ Light Caesar dressing
- ❏ Mandarin oranges in water

Whole grains

- ❏ Whole grain flour
- ❏ Whole wheat flour tortillas
- ❏ Uncooked whole grain oats
- ❏ Whole grain bread
- ❏ Shredded cheese, your choice
- ❏ 90-second whole grain rice
- ❏ Whole wheat spaghetti
- ❏ Whole wheat buns

Protein

- ❏ 1 dozen eggs
- ❏ Turkey bacon
- ❏ Sliced cooked turkey breast
- ❏ Sliced reduced-fat cheese
- ❏ 3 chicken breasts
- ❏ Rotisserie chicken
- ❏ 1 pork chop
- ❏ 1 pound lean ground beef
- ❏ 1 pound ground turkey
- ❏ Small package lean hamburger meat

Dairy

- ❏ ½ gallon reduced-fat milk
- ❏ Butter
- ❏ 2 packages fresh mozzarella (16 oz. packages)
- ❏ 1 container reduced-fat cottage cheese
- ❏ 1 block Parmesan cheese
- ❏ 1 package shredded Monterey Jack cheese
- ❏ Cream cheese

Frozen

- ❏ 1 package strawberries
- ❏ 1 package chopped mango
- ❏ 1 package chopped pineapple

Miscellaneous

- ❏ Cinnamon
- ❏ Pure vanilla extract
- ❏ Minced garlic
- ❏ Dried basil
- ❏ Cumin powder
- ❏ Salt
- ❏ Pepper
- ❏ Garlic powder
- ❏ Dill weed
- ❏ Adobo
- ❏ Smoked paprika
- ❏ Nonstick cooking spray

Week Two

Produce

- ❏ 3 avocados
- ❏ 1 large tomato
- ❏ 1 large container arugula
- ❏ 1 container blueberries
- ❏ 3 bananas
- ❏ 1 container spinach
- ❏ 1 carton strawberries
- ❏ 5 red bell peppers
- ❏ 1 zucchini
- ❏ Salad greens
- ❏ 1 bag radishes
- ❏ 4 red onions
- ❏ 2 cartons cherry tomatoes
- ❏ 6 lemons
- ❏ 1 container raspberries
- ❏ 2 apples

- ❑ 3 heads romaine lettuce
- ❑ 1 package kale
- ❑ 1 cucumber
- ❑ 1 watermelon
- ❑ Snap peas
- ❑ 1 package baby carrots
- ❑ 2 heads broccoli
- ❑ 1 head cauliflower
- ❑ 1 bunch celery
- ❑ 1 container blackberries
- ❑ 1 mango
- ❑ 1 kiwi
- ❑ 2 zucchinis
- ❑ 1 yellow squash
- ❑ 1 carton mushrooms
- ❑ 2 medium yellow onions
- ❑ 1 ½ pounds red potatoes
- ❑ 2 bunches asparagus
- ❑ Fresh parsley
- ❑ Fresh cilantro
- ❑ 1 jalapeño (optional)

Pantry

- ❑ 1 container almonds
- ❑ Ground flaxseed
- ❑ Natural peanut butter
- ❑ Honey
- ❑ Shredded coconut
- ❑ Dried cherries
- ❑ Almond butter
- ❑ Protein pancake mix

- ❑ Pure maple syrup
- ❑ 2 containers salsa
- ❑ 1 container cashews
- ❑ Sugar
- ❑ Dijon mustard
- ❑ Olive oil
- ❑ Shelled sunflower seeds
- ❑ Light mayo
- ❑ 1 croissant
- ❑ Light Caesar salad dressing
- ❑ Dried edamame
- ❑ Dried blueberries
- ❑ 1 container walnuts
- ❑ Packet Italian seasoning
- ❑ Pistachios
- ❑ Hard or soft tortilla shells
- ❑ 90-second whole grain rice
- ❑ Taco seasoning
- ❑ 1 can reduced-sodium black beans
- ❑ Tortilla chips
- ❑ Kalamata olives

Whole grains

- ❑ Whole grain bread
- ❑ Whole grain English muffins
- ❑ 1 pack whole grain tortillas

- ❏ Whole grain crackers
- ❏ 1 package quinoa

Protein

- ❏ 1 dozen eggs
- ❏ Rotisserie chicken
- ❏ 1 pouch or can tuna
- ❏ 8 chicken breasts
- ❏ 1 pound lean ground beef
- ❏ 5 large shrimp, fresh

Dairy

- ❏ 32 oz. container plain Greek yogurt
- ❏ Unsweetened almond milk
- ❏ 16 oz. mozzarella or gorgonzola cheese

- ❏ 4 oz. cheddar cheese
- ❏ 1 container reduced-fat cottage cheese
- ❏ Small block Parmesan cheese
- ❏ Half gallon reduced-fat milk
- ❏ Low-fat sour cream
- ❏ 1 container feta cheese

Frozen

- ❏ Shelled edamame
- ❏ 2 salmon filets (6 oz.)

Miscellaneous

- ❏ Garlic powder
- ❏ Cayenne pepper
- ❏ Chili powder

Week Three

Produce

- ❏ 4 bananas
- ❏ 1 carton strawberries
- ❏ 3 jalapeños
- ❏ 1 carton blueberries
- ❏ 5 apples
- ❏ 4 avocados

- ❏ 1 container spinach
- ❏ 4 large tomatoes
- ❏ 1 large package kale
- ❏ 2 large zucchinis, 2 small zucchinis
- ❏ Alfalfa or broccoli sprouts

- ❑ 2 red peppers
- ❑ 5 red onions
- ❑ 2 heads butter lettuce
- ❑ 3 mangos
- ❑ 1 orange
- ❑ 1 carton blackberries
- ❑ 1 carton raspberries
- ❑ 2 kiwis
- ❑ 1 carton cherry tomatoes
- ❑ Fresh basil
- ❑ Zucchini noodles
- ❑ 1 yellow squash
- ❑ 1 package carrots
- ❑ 1 head broccoli
- ❑ 1 bunch green beans
- ❑ 1 large sweet potato
- ❑ 1 small spaghetti squash
- ❑ 3 green onions
- ❑ Package of brussels sprouts
- ❑ 2 cloves garlic
- ❑ Fresh ginger (1 piece)
- ❑ Fresh cilantro

Pantry

- ❑ Almond butter
- ❑ 1 small bar dark chocolate
- ❑ Chia seeds
- ❑ Honey
- ❑ Natural peanut butter
- ❑ Granola
- ❑ Olive oil
- ❑ 1 can green chilis (7 oz. can)
- ❑ Dried cherries
- ❑ Small container/package walnuts
- ❑ 1 can or pouch of wild-caught salmon or tuna
- ❑ Spinach tortilla shells
- ❑ 1 container hummus
- ❑ 1 can chickpeas
- ❑ Pita bread (2 pieces)
- ❑ Red pepper hummus
- ❑ 1 package of turkey jerky
- ❑ 1 package kale chips
- ❑ 1 small package sliced almonds
- ❑ Balsamic vinaigrette
- ❑ Panko bread crumbs
- ❑ Nutritional yeast
- ❑ 2 cups low-sodium spaghetti sauce
- ❑ 1 package quinoa
- ❑ 1 small can chipotle chilis
- ❑ Fruit cups
- ❑ Hot sauce
- ❑ Red wine vinegar
- ❑ No-salt-added beef broth
- ❑ Cornstarch
- ❑ Low-sodium soy sauce

- ❏ Sesame oil
- ❏ Sesame seeds

Whole grains

- ❏ Dried oats
- ❏ Whole grain cereal
- ❏ Whole grain bread
- ❏ Whole wheat flour
- ❏ Whole wheat tortilla
- ❏ 90-second rice

Protein

- ❏ 2 dozen eggs
- ❏ 1 ½ pound turkey bacon
- ❏ Deli-sliced chicken
- ❏ 2 pounds boneless chicken tenders
- ❏ 3 chicken breasts
- ❏ 1 pound sirloin beef
- ❏ 1 pound lean ground beef
- ❏ 1 pound lean ground turkey
- ❏ 4 grouper or other mild fish

Dairy

- ❏ ½ gallon reduced-fat milk
- ❏ 32 oz. container plain Greek yogurt

- ❏ 1 package sliced cheddar cheese
- ❏ 1 large container fat-free cottage cheese
- ❏ Block of Parmesan cheese
- ❏ 16 oz. fresh mozzarella
- ❏ 1 package cheese sticks
- ❏ 1 container feta cheese
- ❏ Sliced cheese (your choice)
- ❏ Small container sour cream

Frozen

- ❏ Shelled edamame
- ❏ Corn
- ❏ 1 package strawberries
- ❏ Black bean burger
- ❏ 4 cups broccoli florets

Miscellaneous

- ❏ Small container orange juice
- ❏ Paprika
- ❏ Toothpicks
- ❏ Garlic powder
- ❏ Dried thyme
- ❏ Dried oregano
- ❏ Cumin powder

Week Four

Produce

- 2 small green onions
- 1 container mushrooms
- 5 red bell peppers
- 3 tomatoes
- 2 lemons
- 1 container blueberries
- 1 container blackberries
- 2 bananas
- 1 bunch fresh chives
- Fresh basil
- 5 heads broccoli
- 16 oz. container mushrooms
- 2 cucumbers
- Fresh dill
- 1 head romaine
- 1 carton cherry tomatoes
- 3 avocados
- 1 container spinach
- 2 zucchinis
- Shredded lettuce
- 4 red onions
- 1 container strawberries
- 1 package baby carrots
- 1 pear
- 2 kiwis
- 1 lime
- 1 clove garlic
- 1 mixed greens (large container)
- 1 shredded carrots (one bag)
- 1 mango
- 1 bunch watercress
- 2 oranges
- 2 large yellow onions
- Fresh cilantro

Pantry

- 1 cup unsalted cashews
- 1 cup unsalted raw pumpkin seeds
- 1 cup unsalted pecans
- 1 cup unsalted sunflower seeds
- Dried oats
- Natural peanut butter
- Olive oil
- Splenda Brown Sugar Blend
- 1 container almonds
- Blackberry jam
- 1 baguette

- ❏ Unsweet cocoa powder
- ❏ Low-sodium vegetable broth
- ❏ 4 large sun-dried tomatoes
- ❏ Kalamata olives
- ❏ Tzatziki sauce
- ❏ Ranch dressing
- ❏ Vinaigrette dressing
- ❏ Croutons
- ❏ Buffalo sauce
- ❏ Pita bread, one piece
- ❏ Almond butter
- ❏ Dark chocolate almonds, small package
- ❏ Dried blueberries
- ❏ 1 pouch or can tuna
- ❏ Light mayo
- ❏ Fruit cups
- ❏ 1 container salsa
- ❏ Hot sauce
- ❏ 8 corn tortillas (6-inch)
- ❏ 1 can low-sodium garbanzo beans
- ❏ Splenda granulated sweetener
- ❏ Lower-sodium soy sauce
- ❏ Apple cider vinegar
- ❏ 4 cups chicken stock
- ❏ 1 red enchilada sauce (19 oz. can)
- ❏ 1 can fire-roasted tomatoes, diced (14 oz. can)
- ❏ 1 can creamed or sweet corn (14 oz. can)
- ❏ Sugar-free apricot preserves
- ❏ BBQ sauce, your choice of flavor
- ❏ Avocado oil
- ❏ White wine vinegar
- ❏ Small package walnuts
- ❏ Canola oil
- ❏ Salsa or pico de gallo

Whole grains

- ❏ Whole grain English muffins
- ❏ Package of dried farro
- ❏ 90-second whole grain rice
- ❏ Whole grain or nut crackers
- ❏ Whole grain bread
- ❏ Whole grain pasta
- ❏ 12-inch prepackaged whole wheat pizza crust
- ❏ 5 whole wheat flour tortillas (8-inch)

Protein

- ❏ Small container egg substitute or egg whites
- ❏ 2 dozen eggs
- ❏ 2 ½ pounds chicken breast
- ❏ Turkey bacon
- ❏ 2 rotisserie chickens
- ❏ Deli turkey breast, 1 container
- ❏ 1 ¼ pounds firm white fish such as tilapia or halibut
- ❏ ¼ pound salami
- ❏ 4 Alaskan salmon filets (4–6 oz. each)
- ❏ 1 ½ pounds steak

Dairy

- ❏ 32 oz. container plain Greek yogurt
- ❏ ½ gallon reduced-fat milk
- ❏ Shredded Colby Jack cheese
- ❏ 1 container ricotta cheese

- ❏ 1 container goat cheese
- ❏ 1 container feta cheese
- ❏ 3 oz. mozzarella cheese
- ❏ ½ gallon unsweetened almond milk
- ❏ 1 container bleu cheese crumbles
- ❏ Mozzarella cheese sticks
- ❏ 1 package shredded Italian-style cheese

Frozen

- ❏ Shredded hash browns
- ❏ Shelled edamame
- ❏ 1 small package strawberries
- ❏ 1 small package mango

Miscellaneous

- ❏ Pure vanilla extract
- ❏ Paprika
- ❏ Chili powder
- ❏ Ground ginger
- ❏ Dried oregano
- ❏ Sea salt

Menus

Week One

Boldface indicates an item that has a recipe in the next section.

Monday

BREAKFAST

- ¾ cup cooked oatmeal, made with water
- 1 tbsp. sliced almonds
- 1 tbsp. ground flaxseeds
- ¼ cup fresh blueberries

LUNCH

Turkey sandwich on whole wheat bread
- 4 slices of turkey, 1 oz. reduced-fat cheese, lettuce, and onion
- 1 cup raw veggies (broccoli, carrots, tomatoes)
- 2 tbsp. hummus dip

SNACK

- 1 cup strawberries
- 2 oz. fresh mozzarella

DINNER

- **Grilled pork chop, sweet potato, and broccoli**

Tuesday

BREAKFAST

- 1 slice **cinnamon bread**
- 2 scrambled eggs (made with olive oil or nonstick spray)
- 1 tangerine or orange

LUNCH

- **Make-ahead cucumber and onion salad**
- 1 cup mixed seasonal fruit

SNACK

- 1 medium banana
- 1 oz. almonds

DINNER

- **Grilled teriyaki chicken with pineapple, roasted asparagus, and brown rice**

Wednesday

BREAKFAST

Strawberry smoothie
- 1 cup frozen strawberries
- ½ cup frozen mango
- ½ cup frozen pineapple
- 1 cup reduced-fat milk
- Water/ice as needed
- Blend

LUNCH

- **5-minute chicken salad in cucumber boat**
- ½ cup mandarin oranges in water

SNACK

- 1 orange
- 1 oz. pretzels
- 1 hard-boiled egg

DINNER

- **Grilled hamburger** with leaf lettuce, tomato, and onion
- 1 cup of watermelon

Thursday

BREAKFAST

- ¾ cup cooked oatmeal, made with water
- 1 sliced apple and 1 tbsp. raisins
- 2 slices turkey bacon

LUNCH

Blue salad & small baked potato
(with 1 tbsp. butter and dash of pepper)
- 2 cups romaine lettuce, shredded
- ¼ cup tomatoes, chopped
- 2 tbsp. turkey bacon pieces
- 2 tbsp. light bleu cheese dressing

SNACK

- 1 cup reduced-fat cottage cheese
- 1 peach, sliced

DINNER

- **Spaghetti and Caesar salad**

Friday

BREAKFAST

- 1 slice whole wheat toast
- 1 tsp. butter
- 3 scrambled egg whites made with olive oil, salt, and pepper
- 15 grapes

LUNCH

Chicken, rice, and veggie bowl
- In a medium-sized bowl, combine 4 oz. rotisserie chicken, ⅓ cup 90-second whole grain rice, 1 cup chopped veggies your choice, 2 tbsp. dressing

SNACK

- 1 medium graham cracker
- 2 cups watermelon, diced
- 1 oz. almonds or peanuts

DINNER

- **Stuffed green peppers**

1 cup spinach salad
- Chopped spinach
- 1 tsp. slivered almonds
- 5–6 croutons
- Cherry tomatoes
- 1 oz. cheese
- 2 tbsp. choice of dressing

Saturday

BREAKFAST

- **Breakfast burrito**
- 1 apple

LUNCH

- 1 cup carrot sticks
- ½ zucchini, sliced
- 4 tbsp. tzatziki sauce for dipping
- 1 oz. walnuts or almonds

SNACK

- Half slice whole wheat toast
- 1 tbsp. cream cheese
- Sliced fruit on top

DINNER

- **Eggplant parmesan**

Sunday

BREAKFAST

Egg scramble
- Cook ½ cup spinach and mushrooms, add 3 eggs, salt/pepper
- 1 slice whole grain toast
- ½ cup blackberries or raspberries (or your choice of seasonal fresh fruit)

LUNCH

On-the-go tuna lettuce wraps (2 wraps)
- 1 can or pouch tuna (in water), spread evenly on 2 romaine leaves. Top with ¼ avocado each leaf. Top with chopped peppers, cucumber, tomatoes, or desired veggies.
- 1 fruit cup in water

SNACK

- 1 cup baby carrots
- 2 tbsp. ranch dressing or hummus
- 1 banana

DINNER

- **Turkey chili**

Week Two

Boldface indicates an item that has a recipe in the next section.

Monday

BREAKFAST

- ¼ avocado spread on whole grain toast (1 slice), fresh tomato slices, and arugula
- 1 hard-boiled egg

LUNCH

Chicken and veggie wrap
- Spread ¼ avocado on whole grain tortilla shell. Layer 2 oz. of rotisserie chicken, sliced red peppers, sliced zucchini, and salad greens down center of tortilla. Roll tortilla.

SNACK

- 2 cups fresh watermelon
- 2 oz. fresh mozzarella

DINNER

Simple grilled chicken and veggies
- 4 oz. chicken breast, grilled or baked in oven
- 2 cups baked or grilled non-starchy veggies (zucchini, squash, tomatoes, broccoli, asparagus, or peppers)

coated with olive oil, salt, pepper, garlic powder, cayenne pepper (optional)

Tuesday

BREAKFAST

- 1 cup low-fat plain Greek yogurt, topped with
  ½ oz. almonds
  ½ cup blueberries
  1 tsp. ground flaxseed

LUNCH

Fresh salad
- 2 cups arugula, fresh parsley, sliced radishes, red onion, ½ avocado, fresh tomatoes, ¼ cup cashews, ¼ cup gorgonzola or mozzarella cheese, ¼ cup edamame, and sliced red pepper. Served with 2–3 tbsp. **lemon vinaigrette dressing**.

SNACK

Veggies & dip
- Choose 2 cups colorful veggies (snap peas, broccoli, carrot sticks, cauliflower, pepper strips, cucumber, or cherry tomatoes).

Dip
- ½ cup plain Greek yogurt mixed with ranch dressing packet or Italian seasoning packet to taste

DINNER

Quick quinoa and veggies
- Make ½ cup dried quinoa according to directions.
- While cooking, sauté 1 zucchini, ¼ cup mushrooms, 1 yellow onion, 1 red pepper with 2 tbsp. olive oil. Season with salt, pepper, and garlic powder. Mix with quinoa.

Wednesday

BREAKFAST

- 1 slice whole grain bread, toasted
- Top with 1 tbsp. peanut butter, ½ sliced banana, drizzle of honey, shredded coconut, and almond slivers

LUNCH

- 1 cup reduced-fat cottage cheese
- Top with 2 tbsp. shelled sunflower seeds
- 1 cup raspberries

SNACK

Healthy trail mix
- 2 tbsp. dried cherries
- 2 tbsp. almonds
- 2 tbsp. walnuts
- 2 tbsp. dried blueberries

DINNER

- **Chicken, kale, and potato skillet**

Thursday

BREAKFAST

Cherry smoothie
- 1 cup plain Greek yogurt
- 2 tbsp. dried cherries
- 1 banana
- 1 cup unsweetened almond milk
- 1 tbsp. almond butter
- Blend all ingredients. Add liquid to reach desired consistency.

LUNCH

Tuna salad on croissant
- Mix one packet of tuna, 1 tbsp. mayo or avocado, onion, parsley, salt, pepper, paprika, 1 tbsp. Dijon mustard together and top onto a sliced croissant.
- 1 apple

SNACK

Snack box (in a three-compartment container)
- 1 oz. pistachios
- 1 cup raw veggies (carrots, broccoli, or peppers)
- 1 hard-boiled egg

DINNER

Lean ground beef tacos
- 2 tacos (2 oz. lean ground beef in each taco), hard or soft tortilla shells

- Season with taco seasoning, garlic powder, chili powder
- Toppings: spinach, tomato, red onion, salsa, 2 tbsp. plain Greek yogurt

Friday

BREAKFAST

- **Breakfast egg sandwich**
- 1 cup blueberries

LUNCH

- 8 whole grain crackers
- 2 oz. low-fat cheddar cheese
- 2 hard-boiled eggs
- 1 piece of fruit, your choice

SNACK

- 1 sliced apple with 2 tbsp. peanut butter. Topped with ¼ cup mixture of dried cherries, blueberries, and crushed almonds.

DINNER

6 oz. salmon & 1 cup asparagus
- Place asparagus and fish in pan with 1 tbsp. olive oil.
- Season with salt, pepper, garlic powder.
- Bake, uncovered, at 425° for 15–20 minutes or until fish flakes easily with a fork.

- Serve with asparagus and ½ cup cooked instant brown rice.

Saturday

BREAKFAST

- Three 4-inch protein pancakes or waffles (make according to package)
- Top with ½ cup berries
- 1 tsp. pure maple syrup

LUNCH

- **5-minute chicken Caesar salad wrap**

SNACK

- 1 cup carrot and celery sticks
- 2 tbsp. peanut butter
- ½ cup fresh blackberries or raspberries

DINNER

Tex Mex salad
- 3 oz. of grilled chicken or beef on top of 2 cups shredded romaine lettuce. Top with 1 oz. cheddar cheese, tomatoes, salsa, ¼ cup rinsed black beans, taco seasoning, ¼ avocado, 1 tbsp. sour cream, jalapeño (optional), red onion, and 6 crushed tortilla chips.

Sunday

BREAKFAST

Mexican egg scramble
- Sauté ½ red pepper, 2 eggs, and 2 tbsp. salsa. Cheese optional.
- Serve with toast or 1 warm tortilla.

LUNCH

Kale & veggie salad
- 2 cups of fresh kale topped with ½ cup dried edamame, ½ cup cooked quinoa, ½ cup chopped veggies (tomato, cucumber, and red pepper), and 2 tbsp. choice of vinaigrette

SNACK

Mixed fruit
- Mix ¼ banana sliced, ¼ cup blackberries, ¼ chopped fresh mango, and 1 kiwi. Squeeze one fresh lemon on top.
- 1 oz. fresh mozzarella or 6 oz. low-fat milk

DINNER

- **Mediterranean shrimp**

Week Three

Boldface indicates an item that has a recipe in the next section.

Monday

BREAKFAST

Overnight oats
- Layer ingredients in your choice of container.
- ½ cup dried oats, ½ cup low-fat milk, ¼ cup plain yogurt, 1 tablespoon almond butter, ½ banana, sliced, 1 tsp. chopped dark chocolate, 1 tsp. chia seeds. Refrigerate overnight.

LUNCH

Simple salad
- 3 cups spinach
- 1 oz. fresh mozzarella
- 2 tbsp. dried cherries
- ½ cup chopped tomatoes
- 2 tbsp. oil & vinegar vinaigrette
- Top with 2 tbsp. walnuts & 1 wild-caught tuna or salmon pouch

SNACK

Smoothie
- Blend ½ cup ice, 6 oz. plain Greek yogurt, ½ banana, ½ mango, ½ cup frozen strawberries, and ¼ cup orange juice. Add liquid (water) to reach desired consistency.

DINNER

- **Healthy baked chicken tenders with spicy honey mustard sauce**
- Serve with mixed non-starchy veggies (zucchini, broccoli, carrots, cauliflower, peppers, squash, green beans, etc.)

Tuesday

BREAKFAST

- **Breakfast egg cups**
- ½ cup seasonal fruit

LUNCH

- 1 cup kale chips (homemade or store bought)
- 1 cheese stick
- 1 piece of fruit

SNACK

Avocado deviled eggs
- 2 hard-boiled eggs (use egg yolk from one egg and 2 tbsp. avocado). Smash together and add paprika, salt, pepper, and cayenne pepper (optional). Fill eggs.
- 1 orange

DINNER

Black bean burger and fries
- 1 black bean burger (cook according to package)
- Cut whole grain bread into circles for bun
- 1 cup **sweet potato fries**
- Top with tomato slice, spinach, and sliced onion

Wednesday

BREAKFAST

Cereal and fruit
- ¾ cup whole grain cereal
- ½ sliced banana
- ¼ cup blueberries
- 1 cup reduced-fat milk

LUNCH

Hummus wrap
- 1 spinach tortilla shell
- Spread 2 tbsp. hummus on shell.
- Add spinach, tomato, zucchini, and fresh alfalfa or broccoli sprouts.

SNACK

Mixed fruit and cottage cheese
- ¼ cup blackberries, ¼ cup raspberries, and 1 kiwi sliced on top of 1 cup cottage cheese

DINNER

- **Spaghetti squash and meatballs**
- 1 slice whole grain bread or roll, 1 tsp. butter

Thursday

BREAKFAST

- 1 cup plain Greek yogurt
- 2 tsp. honey
- 1 tbsp. almond or peanut butter
- ½ banana

LUNCH

Edamame salad
- Mix 1 cup frozen edamame (thawed), 1 chopped red pepper, ½ small red onion, 1 tomato chopped, ¼ avocado, ¼ cup feta cheese, ¼ cup frozen corn (thawed), 2 tbsp. oil & vinegar vinaigrette

SNACK

- 2 oz. turkey jerky
- 1 apple

DINNER

- **Turkey burger** on whole grain bun
- 1 cup fresh fruit

Friday

BREAKFAST

- 1 large apple, sliced
- 2 tbsp. peanut butter
- 1 tsp. granola on top

LUNCH

Easy pita sandwich #1
- Stuff pita with:
    1 tbsp. red pepper hummus
    ¼ cup chickpeas
    1 oz. feta cheese
    Butter lettuce
    Red onion

SNACK

Yogurt and almond parfait
- In a small jar, layer ½ cup fruit cut into ½-inch cubes (kiwis, mangos, and pineapples) with ¼ cup plain low-fat Greek yogurt. Top with 1 tbsp. toasted sliced almonds.

DINNER

- **Baked fish filets**
- 1 cup roasted brussels sprouts (preheat oven at 400°F, cut in half and coat with olive oil, bake for 30 minutes; top with salt and pepper)
- ⅓ cup whole grain rice made with 1 tsp. olive oil and seasonings

Saturday

BREAKFAST

- 1 slice whole grain toast, topped with ¼ avocado, 1 slice turkey bacon, and 1 sunny-side up egg. Add salt/pepper to taste.
- 1 cup seasonal fruit

LUNCH

Easy pita sandwich #2
- Stuff pita with:
    Chopped kale
    2 tbsp. crushed almonds
    Chopped apples
    ¼ avocado
    Choice of vinaigrette dressing

SNACK

Fruit wrap
- Spread 2 tbsp. peanut butter on a whole wheat tortilla. Top with sliced strawberries, bananas, or kiwi; roll and eat!

DINNER

- **Chicken and mango salsa lettuce wraps**
- 2–3 wraps

Sunday

BREAKFAST

- **Southwest breakfast quiche**
- 2 pieces

LUNCH

Roasted chicken sandwich with fruit
- Roasted deli-sliced chicken on whole grain bread (3 slices of nitrite-free chicken breast), 1 oz. cheese, toppings (lettuce, tomato, onion, etc.), 1 tbsp. mustard or mayo
- 1 medium fruit

SNACK

Mini Caprese skewers
- Take 5–7 toothpicks and fill with tomatoes, mozzarella, basil, and drizzle with balsamic vinaigrette.

DINNER

- **Beef and broccoli over zucchini noodles**

Week Four

Boldface indicates an item that has a recipe in the next section.

Monday

BREAKFAST

- ¼ cup **Power Granola**
- ¾ cup plain Greek yogurt

LUNCH

Mediterranean chicken farro bowl
- Scoop ½ cup cooked farro into a bowl. Top with 4 oz. grilled chicken slices, 1 oz. feta cheese, ¼ cup chopped cucumber, 5 kalamata olives, 1 tbsp. tzatziki sauce, a squeeze of a lemon, and freshly chopped dill.

SNACK

- 1 cup sliced, fresh zucchini
- 2 oz. roasted, salted almonds

DINNER

- **Spicy fish tacos**
- 2 tacos

Tuesday

BREAKFAST

- **Whole wheat breakfast pizzas**

LUNCH

BLT salad
- 2 cups romaine lettuce
- 2 tbsp. crispy turkey bacon
- ¼ cup cherry tomatoes
- 1 oz. mozzarella cheese
- ¼ avocado
- 2 tbsp. ranch dressing

SNACK

Three-compartment container
- Turkey and cheese rollups (2 oz. turkey and 2 oz. cheese)
- pita bread (½ pita)
- ½ cup baby carrots

DINNER

Easy chickpea pasta salad
- Make whole grain pasta (2 oz. dry), add ½ cup broccoli, ¼ cup bell peppers, 1 oz. mozzarella cheese, ¼ cup garbanzo beans, ¼ cup fresh sliced tomatoes, red onion, 1 oz. salami, choice of dressing (2 tbsp.)

Wednesday

BREAKFAST

Blueberry lemon yogurt parfait
- 1 cup nonfat plain Greek yogurt, zest of 1 lemon, ½ tsp. pure vanilla extract, ¾ cup fresh blueberries, ¼ cup sliced almonds

LUNCH

Rice and edamame salad
- Mix ½ cup 90-second whole grain rice, 1 tomato, ½ cup spinach, ½ cup broccoli, ¼ cup edamame, ½ cup red peppers, ⅛ zucchini, 1 oz. mozzarella cheese, and 3 tbsp. vinaigrette dressing.

SNACK

Three-compartment container
- Sliced pear
- 1 tbsp. almond butter
- 8 whole grain crackers or nut crackers

DINNER

- **Baked teriyaki chicken**
- Serve over ⅓ cup whole grain rice
- 1 cup steamed broccoli

Thursday

BREAKFAST

Ricotta and blackberry jam crostini
- 3 small slices of toasted baguette. Add 1 tsp. ricotta to each. Top with blackberry jam and fresh blackberries.
- 1 cup reduced-fat milk

LUNCH

Fruit and almond smoothie
- 1 cup frozen strawberries and mango
- ½ cup plain Greek yogurt
- 1 cup unsweetened almond milk

SNACK

Three-compartment container
- Raw broccoli (larger section)
- 2 hard-boiled eggs
- 1 cheese stick

DINNER

- **5-ingredient chicken tortilla soup**
- Serve with sautéed bell peppers (2 peppers). Cut into strips, sauté with 1 tbsp. olive oil, salt, pepper, and garlic powder.

Friday

BREAKFAST

Peanut butter banana smoothie
- 1 cup reduced-fat milk
- 1 frozen banana
- 2 tbsp. peanut butter
- 1 tbsp. cocoa powder, unsweetened

LUNCH

Buffalo chicken bowl
- Make ahead 4 oz. shredded chicken or rotisserie chicken, and add 3 tbsp. buffalo sauce.
- Top with shredded lettuce, 1 hard-boiled egg, 1 oz. blue cheese crumbles, diced red onions, tomatoes, ¼ avocado, and ½ cup croutons.

SNACK

Three-compartment container
- Sliced kiwi and strawberries (larger section)
- Nonfat plain Geek yogurt (6–8 oz.)
- 8 dark chocolate almonds

DINNER

- **BBQ chicken pizza**
- 2 slices
- Serve with side mixed green salad

Saturday

BREAKFAST

- **Savory Mediterranean oats**

LUNCH

- 1 mozzarella cheese stick
- 1 cup strawberries
- 2 hard-boiled eggs

SNACK

Three-compartment container
- ½ peanut butter sandwich (larger section)
- Dried blueberries (¼ cup)
- Almonds (1 oz.)

DINNER

- **Alaskan salmon with orange watercress**
- ½ fresh mango cut into cubes

Sunday

BREAKFAST

- **Mushroom and broccoli frittata**

LUNCH

Smoothie lunch bowl
- ½ cup unsweetened almond milk, 1 frozen banana, 1 cup baby spinach, 1 cup frozen mixed fruit, ¼ cup plain Greek yogurt
- Combine all ingredients in a blender. Purée until smooth. Sprinkle with ¼ cup of **Power Granola**.

SNACK

Tuna salad
- 1 packet of tuna, 1 tbsp. mayo or avocado, onion, paprika, salt, pepper, 3 crushed crackers
- 1 fruit cup, in water

DINNER

- **Beef fajitas**
- Serve with side mixed green salad

Recipes

Week One

CINNAMON BREAD

2 cups bread flour
1 cup whole wheat flour
½ cup of Splenda Brown
  Sugar Blend
1 (5.1 ounce) package
  instant sugar-free vanilla
  pudding mix
½ tsp. baking soda
1 ½ tsp. baking powder
½ tsp. salt

2 tsp. ground cinnamon
1 ½ cups skim milk
½ cup canola oil
½ cup unsweetened
  applesauce
1 whole egg
1 tsp. vanilla
2 tbsp. cinnamon sucralose
  blend

- Preheat oven to 350°F. Spray 2 loaf pans with nonstick cooking spray.
- Sprinkle bottom of pans with 1 tbsp. cinnamon sucralose blend.
- In a large bowl, combine flours, sugar, pudding mix, baking soda, baking powder, salt, and cinnamon. In a separate bowl, combine the milk, oil, applesauce, eggs, and vanilla.
- Stir milk mixture into dry mixture until smooth. Divide the batter and pour evenly into the 2 pans.
- Sprinkle tops of batter with remaining cinnamon sucralose blend.
- Bake 1 hour or until a toothpick inserted in the center comes out clean.

24 servings

BREAKFAST BURRITO

1 10" whole wheat flour
  tortilla
2 egg whites, scrambled

2 tbsp. shredded cheese
1 tbsp. turkey bacon pieces

- Separate egg yolks from egg whites and scramble in skillet sprayed with nonstick cooking spray. Add turkey bacon pieces while scrambling eggs. Heat tortilla in microwave for 10 seconds. Fill tortilla with egg and sprinkle with cheese. Serve warm.

1 serving

MAKE-AHEAD CUCUMBER AND ONION SALAD

1 large cucumber,
  thinly sliced
1 onion, thinly sliced
½ cup white vinegar

⅓ cup water
¼ tsp. salt
Dash of pepper
¼ tsp. celery seed

- Slice cucumbers and onions into glass bowl. Mix remaining ingredients in small bowl and pour over cucumbers and onions. Cover and refrigerate 3 hours. Drain and serve.

3–4 servings

5-MINUTE CHICKEN SALAD IN CUCUMBER BOAT

2 cups cooked chicken,
shredded
2 celery stalks, chopped

⅓ cup light mayo
1 tbsp. dill weed
1 large cucumber

- Combine shredded, cooked chicken with ingredients
  and mix well. Wash and peel cucumber and slice in
  half, creating two long halves.
- Using a spoon, carve out seeds to create a cucumber
  boat. Fill each cucumber with chicken salad.

4 servings of ¾ cup

GRILLED PORK CHOP, SWEET POTATO, AND BROCCOLI

3 oz. grilled pork chop
5 oz. baked sweet potato
½ cup steamed broccoli

Salt and pepper, to taste
1 tsp. brown sugar
Cinnamon, to taste

- Season pork chop with a dash of salt and pepper. Grill
  or broil for 6–8 minutes on both sides or until juices
  run clear.

1 serving

Baked sweet potato
- Preheat oven to 425°F. Poke holes in sweet potato.
  Cook for 45 minutes until done.
- Add brown sugar and cinnamon.

1 serving

Steamed broccoli
- Clean and chop broccoli. Place in steamer and cook for 5 minutes.

1 serving

GRILLED TERIYAKI CHICKEN WITH PINEAPPLE, ROASTED ASPARAGUS, AND BROWN RICE

3 oz. skinless boneless
chicken breast
1 tbsp. teriyaki sauce
Salt and pepper, to taste

1 bunch of asparagus
2 tbsp. olive oil
90-second microwave rice
1 pineapple ring

For Chicken
- In a resealable plastic bag, marinate 3 oz. skinless boneless chicken breast in 1 tbsp. teriyaki sauce for 1 hour. Grill on high heat and grill for 6–8 minutes on each side or until juices run clear when pierced with a fork.
- Grill pineapple ring on both sides until warmed through.

1 serving

For Asparagus
- Wash 20 spears of fresh asparagus. Hold spear on both ends and bend to break edible portion from inedible portion. Place in baking dish and coat with 2 tbsp. olive oil. Sprinkle with ⅛ tsp. salt and ¼ tsp. black pepper.
- Roast at 400°F for 12–15 minutes. Also could be cooked on the grill.

4 servings of 5 spears

For Rice
- Use 90-second brown rice in microwave pouch.

2.5 servings of ¾ cup

GRILLED HAMBURGER

2 oz. lean hamburger
Seasonings of choice
1 whole wheat bun

Leaf lettuce
1 slice tomato
Slice of onion

- Grill hamburger on medium-high heat until desired doneness. Add toppings and serve with watermelon.

1 serving

SPAGHETTI AND CAESAR SALAD

1 cup cooked whole wheat
  spaghetti
¼ cup marinara sauce
Caesar salad
2 cups romaine lettuce,
  shredded

1 tbsp. Parmesan cheese,
  shredded
2 tbsp. light Caesar
  dressing

- Cook pasta according to directions and add sauce. Add any desired seasonings.
- Serve with one salad.

1 serving

STUFFED GREEN PEPPERS

6 large green peppers
5 cups boiling water
1 lb. 95% lean ground
   beef
2 tbsp. onion, chopped

1 tsp. salt
⅛ tsp. garlic salt
1 cup cooked rice
2 cups spaghetti sauce
1 tsp. fresh-cut basil

- Preheat oven to 350°F.
- Slice off top of green pepper and clean inside.
- Wash and put into boiling water for 5 minutes and then drain.
- Cook beef and onion until onion is tender. Drain off fat. Stir in salt, garlic salt, rice, and 1 cup spaghetti sauce.
- Lightly stuff peppers with ½ cup of beef mixture. Stand upright in ungreased baking dish. Pour remaining spaghetti sauce over the peppers. Cover and bake 45 minutes. Top with fresh basil.

6 servings

EGGPLANT PARMESAN

3 eggplants, peeled and
   thinly sliced
2 eggs, beaten
4 cups Italian-seasoned
   bread crumbs
6 cups spaghetti sauce,
   divided

1 (16 oz.) package
   mozzarella cheese,
   shredded and
   divided
½ cup grated Parmesan
   cheese, divided
½ teaspoon dried basil

- Preheat oven to 350°F.

- Dip eggplant slices in egg, then in bread crumbs. Place in a single layer on a baking sheet. Bake in preheated oven for 5 minutes on each side.
- In a 9- by 13-inch baking dish, spread spaghetti sauce to cover the bottom. Place a layer of eggplant slices in the sauce. Sprinkle with mozzarella and Parmesan cheeses. Repeat with remaining ingredients, ending with the cheeses. Sprinkle basil on top.
- Bake in preheated oven for 35 minutes, or until golden brown.

6–8 servings

TURKEY CHILI

2 tbsp. extra-virgin olive oil

1 green bell pepper, chopped

1 small onion, finely chopped

2 tbsp. minced garlic

1 lb. ground turkey

1 ½ teaspoons ground cumin

All-purpose seasoning with pepper, to taste

2 (15 oz.) cans low-sodium red kidney beans, drained

2 (8 oz.) cans tomato sauce

1 cup water

1 chipotle chile, finely chopped from 1 can (7 oz.) chipotle chiles

¼ cup shredded Monterey Jack cheese

1 avocado, chopped

Coarsely chopped fresh cilantro

- Heat oil in medium pot over medium heat. Stir in peppers, onions, and garlic; cook until tender, 5–7 minutes. Add turkey, cumin, and All-purpose seasoning. Cook, breaking up turkey with spoon, until browned, about 5 minutes.

• Stir in beans, tomato sauce, water, and chipotle; bring liquid to boil. Reduce heat. Simmer until chili thickens and flavors come together, about 10 minutes.

• Divide chili among serving bowls. Top with cheese, avocado, and cilantro.

4 servings

WEEK ONE AVERAGE NUTRITIONAL BREAKDOWN	
49% CARBS, 19% PROTEIN, 32% FAT	
Calories: 1,454	Fat: 44g
Carbohydrates: 164g	Fiber: 29g
Protein: 72g	Added sugar: 0g

Week Two

BREAKFAST EGG SANDWICH

1 whole grain English
  muffin
Handful spinach
1 tomato slice

1 oz. mozzarella
  cheese
1 whole egg
1 egg white

• Scramble egg in nonstick pan over medium-high heat.
• Place cheese on one part of English muffin and top with scrambled egg, spinach, and tomato. Top with muffin and serve.

1 serving

LEMON VINAIGRETTE DRESSING

½ tsp. finely grated lemon zest

2 tbsp. freshly squeezed lemon juice

1 tsp. sugar

½ tsp. Dijon mustard

¼ tsp. fine sea salt, or to taste

3–4 tbsp. extra-virgin olive oil

Freshly ground black pepper, to taste

• Whisk all ingredients together for thirty seconds and mix well.

CHICKEN, KALE, AND POTATO SKILLET DINNER

3 tbsp. olive oil

1 ½ pounds red potatoes, cut in half and boiled in salted water until fork tender

Salt and pepper, to taste

2 tsp. dried thyme

6 chicken breasts, thinly sliced

1 onion, medium, thinly sliced

1 tbsp. garlic, minced

1 bunch curly kale, stems removed and roughly chopped

1 lemon, optional

• Heat 2 tbsp. olive oil in a large 15-inch skillet over medium-high heat. Add potatoes (cut side down) and cook without stirring until they begin to turn golden brown. Stir and continue cooking until all sides are crispy, about 5–7 minutes. Depending on the size of your pan, you may have to do this in a few batches. Season potatoes with salt, pepper, and thyme.

- Add another tbsp. of olive oil and the chicken to the potatoes. Cook until both sides of chicken are done, about 6 minutes each side, or internal temperature is 165 degrees. Once done, add onions and cook until just tender, stirring often, about 5 minutes.
- Reduce heat to medium and add the garlic, stirring until fragrant, about one minute. Add the kale. Stir often and cooking until the kale is wilted, about 3 minutes.
- Squeeze a lemon over the top of the dish and serve.

6 servings

MEDITERRANEAN SHRIMP

5 large shrimp, peeled
1 ½ tbsp. olive oil, divided
2 tsp. minced garlic
1 pinch sea salt and ground
    black pepper, to taste
2 tsp. each, paprika and
    oregano

1 whole lemon, juiced
1 bunch fresh asparagus
1 whole read onion, sliced
¼ cup feta cheese
¼ cup kalamata olives
⅓ cup fresh cilantro or
    parsley

- Preheat oven to 450° F.
- In a large bowl season the shrimp with 1 tbsp. olive oil, garlic, salt, black pepper, paprika, oregano, and juice from lemon.
- Trim and wash the asparagus, then lay them flat on the baking sheet. Season with ½ tbsp. olive oil. Place seasoned shrimp on top of asparagus and top with sliced red onions.
- Bake for 10 minutes in the middle rack. Shrimp is cooked when the edges start to turn golden brown.

- Remove shrimp from oven and top with feta, olives, and fresh cilantro or parsley. Drizzle with remaining olive oil and serve.

1 serving

5-MINUTE CHICKEN CAESAR SALAD LUNCH WRAP

1 ½ cup cooked chicken, diced

3 tbsp. light Caesar salad dressing

3 tbsp. Parmesan cheese, freshly shredded

4 cups chopped romaine lettuce

4 tortillas (10-inch, low-carb)

- In a medium bowl, mix together all the ingredients except for the tortillas. Coat the salad evenly with the dressing.
- Spread 1 heaping cup of the chicken salad mixture onto the tortilla. Fold the left and right sides of the wrap in until they touch and roll from the bottom to make a wrap.
- Repeat procedure for remaining 3 wraps.

4 servings

WEEK TWO AVERAGE NUTRITIONAL BREAKDOWN	
38% CARBS, 22% PROTEIN, 40% FAT	
Calories: 1,466	Fat: 62g
Carbohydrates: 139g	Fiber: 34g
Protein: 81g	Added sugar: 1g

Week Three

BREAKFAST EGG CUPS

12 eggs
½ cup milk
1 tsp. salt
½ tsp. pepper
1 lb. cooked bacon,
  chopped (optional)

2 cups cheddar cheese,
  shredded
2 jalapeños, seeded and
  diced
Fresh cilantro, optional

- Preheat oven to 350°F. In a large mixing bowl, whisk together eggs, milk, salt, and pepper.
- Grease a 12-cup muffin tin. Evenly disperse half of the bacon, cheese, and jalapeños into cups. Pour egg mixture into the cups, filling ½ full. Top with remaining ingredients (evenly dispersed among the pan).
- Bake on center rack for 20–25 minutes. Top with fresh cilantro and serve!

Notes:
- Breakfast egg cups can be stored in an airtight container for up to 5 days. To reheat, microwave for 1 minute or place in a preheated oven at 400°F for 5 minutes.

12 servings

SOUTHWEST BREAKFAST QUICHE

3 eggs

¼ cup whole wheat flour

½ tsp. baking powder

½ cup egg whites or egg substitute

¼ cup skim milk

1 (7 oz.) can green chilis

1 cup fat-free cottage cheese (whipped in a food processor until smooth)

1 cup reduced-fat shredded cheddar cheese

- Preheat oven to 400° F. Coat a 9-inch round or square baking dish with canola cooking spray; set aside.
- In mixer bowl, combine eggs, flour, and baking powder, and beat until blended. Add egg whites and milk and beat until smooth. On low speed, beat in green chilis, cottage cheese, and shredded cheese.
- Pour mixture into prepared dish and bake for 15 minutes. Reduce heat to 350°F and bake for about 25 minutes more (until quiche is firm in the center and top is golden brown). Cut into 6 equal slices and serve as is or top with salsa, avocado, or plain Greek yogurt.

6 servings

HEALTHY BAKED CHICKEN TENDERS WITH SPICY HONEY MUSTARD SAUCE

For the Chicken Tenders

1 egg

½ cup sour cream

1–2 lb. boneless chicken tenders

½ cup panko bread crumbs

½ cup nutritional yeast

½ tsp. paprika

½ tsp. garlic powder

½ tsp. sea salt

½ tsp. black pepper

½ tsp. thyme

½ tsp. Italian seasoning

For the Spicy Honey Mustard

1 cup Dijon mustard

½ cup honey

½ cup mayonnaise

¼ tsp. ground cayenne

Pinch of sea salt and pepper, to taste

Pinch of smoked paprika

- Preheat oven to 400°F and spray baking sheets with nonstick cooking spray.
- In a small bowl, whisk together egg and sour cream and set aside.
- In another small bowl, mix together the bread crumbs, nutritional yeast, paprika, garlic powder, salt, pepper, thyme, and Italian seasoning. Mix until well blended, then add to a shallow bowl or large plate.
- One by one, dip chicken tenders into sour cream/egg mixture, then coat completely with seasoning bread crumb mixture, then place on baking sheet. Repeat with all chicken tenders until fully covered.
- Bake chicken tenders for 25 minutes, flipping once halfway through, or until internal temperature reads 165°F.
- While chicken tenders are cooking, mix together all honey mustard ingredients until smooth and adjust seasonings to taste (for more sweetness, add more honey, for more mustard taste, add more mustard, etc.).
- Once chicken tenders have cooled, dip in honey mustard and enjoy!

4 servings

SWEET POTATO FRIES

1 large sweet potato, peeled
1 tbsp. olive oil
1 tsp. garlic powder

1 tsp. paprika
¼ tsp. salt
½ tsp. black pepper

- Heat the oven to 400°F.
- Cut the sweet potatoes into sticks ¼–½ inch wide and 3 inches long and toss them with the oil.
- Mix the spices, salt, and pepper in a small bowl, and toss them with the sweet potatoes. Spread them out on 2 rimmed baking sheets.
- Bake until brown and crisp on the bottom, about 15 minutes, then flip and cook until the other side is crisp, about 10 minutes. Serve hot.

2 servings

SPAGHETTI SQUASH AND MEATBALLS

1 small spaghetti squash
1 lb. very lean ground beef (95% lean)
¼ cup plain bread crumbs
3 tbsp. grated, reduced-fat Parmesan cheese (divided)
¾ cup water (plus extra for cooking squash, divided)

2 tbsp. chopped fresh parsley
1 egg
1 tsp. garlic powder
½ tsp. black pepper
2 cups low-sodium spaghetti sauce

- Put the whole squash in a soup pot with 1 inch water. Bring to a boil over high heat, cover, and cook 25–30 minutes, or until tender when pierced with a knife. Remove squash to a cutting board and allow to cool slightly. Cut squash in half lengthwise; remove and discard seeds with a spoon. Scrape inside of squash with a fork, shredding into noodle-like strands. Cover to keep warm.

- Meanwhile, in a large bowl, combine ground beef, bread crumbs, 2 tablespoons Parmesan cheese, ¼ cup water, parsley, egg, garlic powder, and pepper; gently mix until well combined. Form mixture into 8 equal-size meatballs.
- Coat a large skillet with cooking spray. Cook meatballs over medium heat 8–10 minutes or until browned, turning them occasionally. Add spaghetti sauce and remaining ½ cup water. Cover and cook 10–15 minutes or until meatballs are no longer pink in center.
- Serve the spaghetti squash topped with sauce and meatballs. Sprinkle with remaining 1 tablespoon Parmesan cheese just before serving.

4 servings

TURKEY BURGER

1 lb. lean ground turkey or chicken

⅓ cup quinoa (cooked, golden or red)

3 green onions, minced

½ cup kale, chopped

2 tbsp. extra-virgin olive oil

½ tsp. cumin

1 tsp. dried oregano

1 tsp. chili powder

1 chipotle chili in adobo, minced (optional)

- In a large bowl, combine all ingredients and mix well to distribute. Shape into 6 patties.
- Preheat grill to medium high and place burgers on grill grate. Cook under direct heat (with the grill closed) for 5–6 minutes per side until cooked through to doneness.

1 serving

BAKED FISH FILETS

Nonstick cooking spray
4 grouper or other mild
   fish fillets (4 oz. each,
   rinsed and patted dry)
3 tbsp. olive oil
2 tbsp. fresh parsley, finely
   chopped

1 tsp. Dijon mustard
   (lowest sodium available)
¼ tsp. dried thyme,
   crumbled
¼ tsp. red-hot pepper
   sauce
⅛ tsp. salt

- Preheat the oven to 350°F. Lightly spray a baking sheet with cooking spray.
- Place the fish on the baking sheet. Bake for 18–20 minutes, or until the fish flakes easily when tested with a fork.
- Meanwhile, in a small bowl, stir together the remaining ingredients.
- Drizzle olive oil mixture over the fish.

4 servings

CHICKEN AND MANGO SALSA LETTUCE WRAPS

Salt, pepper, chili powder, garlic powder, and cayenne pepper, to taste

3 chicken breasts

1 mango (peeled, diced, and hard center squeezed to release 1 tbsp. juice)

½ small red onion, diced

1 medium jalapeño pepper, seeded and minced

1 large red bell pepper, seeded and diced

2 tbsp. red wine vinegar

1 tbsp. olive oil

1 tbsp. honey or 2 packets artificial sweetener

10 butter lettuce (butter lettuce leaves) or romaine lettuce

- Thinly slice chicken breasts. Season with salt, pepper, chili powder, garlic powder, and cayenne pepper. Add olive oil and chicken to skillet. Cook until done (about 6 minutes each side or internal chicken temperature of 165°F).
- Combine all ingredients in a medium-sized bowl except lettuce.
- Assemble wraps.
- If using butter lettuce leaves, arrange them on a large plate and fill each one with ¼ cup of salad mixture.

5 servings

BEEF AND BROCCOLI OVER ZUCCHINI NOODLES

1 cup no-salt-added beef broth

1 tbsp. cornstarch

2 tbsp. lower-sodium soy sauce

2 cloves garlic, minced

1 tbsp. minced fresh ginger
Nonstick cooking spray
2 tsp. toasted sesame oil
1 medium onion, sliced
1 lb. sirloin beef, sliced
4 cups fresh or frozen
broccoli florets

2 small zucchinis (spiral
into noodles, or 4 cups
prepared zucchini
noodles)
2 tbsp. sesame seeds

- In a small bowl, whisk together the broth, cornstarch, soy sauce, garlic, and ginger. Set aside.
- Spray large sauté pan or wok with cooking spray, add sesame oil, and place over high heat.
- Add the onion and stir-fry 2 minutes. Add the beef and stir-fry 3 more minutes.
- Add the broccoli and spiraled zucchini and stir-fry 3 more minutes.
- Add the broth mixture and bring to a boil, scraping the bottom of the pan to loosen any brown bits. Reduce heat and simmer 2 minutes.
- Stir in sesame seeds and serve.

4 servings

WEEK THREE AVERAGE NUTRITIONAL BREAKDOWN	
41% CARBS, 21% PROTEIN, 38% FAT	
Calories: 1,466	Fat: 53g
Carbohydrates: 149g	Fiber: 30g
Protein: 77g	Added sugar: 3g

Week Four

POWER GRANOLA

1 cup unsalted cashews, chopped

1 cup unsalted raw pumpkin seeds (pepitas)

1 cup unsalted pecans, chopped

1 cup unsalted sunflower seeds

1 cup old-fashioned rolled oats (not quick cooking)

¼ cup peanut butter

¼ cup olive oil

¼ cup Splenda Brown Sugar Blend

- Preheat the oven to 300°F.
- Line a baking sheet with parchment paper or foil. Coat with nonstick cooking spray and set aside.
- In a bowl, combine cashews, pumpkin seeds, pecans, sunflower seeds, and oats. Set aside.
- In the microwave, melt peanut butter, oil, and Splenda Brown Sugar together. Stir to combine.
- Pour peanut butter mixture over oat mixture and stir to coat.
- Spread granola in a packed, single layer onto prepared baking sheet. Bake for 40–45 minutes, stirring every 10 minutes to ensure even browning.
- Remove from oven and let cool completely. Break up granola and store in an airtight container.

4–6 servings

WHOLE WHEAT BREAKFAST PIZZAS

1 tsp. butter

2 small green onions, finely chopped

2 small button mushrooms, sliced

½ red bell pepper, diced

½ cup egg substitute

2 tbsp. milk (fat-free)

1 whole grain English muffins (split in half)

¼ cup Colby and Monterey Jack cheese mixture (low-fat, shredded)

1 small tomato, seeded and chopped

- Preheat the oven to 375°F.
- In a small nonstick skillet, heat the butter over medium heat until melted, swirling to coat the bottom. Cook the green onions, mushrooms, and bell pepper over medium-high heat for 3 minutes, or until tender, stirring frequently.
- In a small bowl, whisk together the egg substitute and milk. Pour over the vegetables. Reduce the heat to medium. Cook without stirring until the mixture begins to set on the bottom and around the edge. As it sets, push the mixture toward the center of the skillet and tilt the skillet so the uncooked portion flows to the edge and all the egg substitute is fully cooked, 3–4 minutes. (A rubber scraper works well for this.)
- Put the English muffin halves with the cut side up on a baking sheet. Sprinkle each with 1 tbsp. Colby and Monterey Jack mixture. Spoon the egg mixture over the cheese. Top with the remaining cheese. Sprinkle with the tomato.
- Bake for 5–8 minutes, or until the cheese is melted.

2 servings

SAVORY MEDITERRANEAN OATS

1 cup low-sodium
vegetable broth
4 large sun-dried tomatoes
(halves, not oil-packed,
thinly sliced, do not
rehydrate)
Pinch sea salt, to taste
Freshly ground black
pepper, to taste
½ cup old-fashioned rolled
oats

1 tbsp. fresh chives,
minced
3 tbsp. plain nonfat Greek
yogurt (fat-free)
1 tbsp. fresh basil, thinly
sliced
1 tbsp. soft goat cheese,
crumbled

- Bring the broth, sun-dried tomatoes, salt, and pepper
  to a boil in a small saucepan.
- Stir in the oats and chives and reduce heat to
  medium. Stir, until the oats are fully cooked, about 5
  minutes. Remove from the heat and stir in the yogurt.
- Transfer to a bowl, sprinkle with the basil and goat
  cheese, and serve.

1 serving

MUSHROOM AND BROCCOLI FRITTATA

Nonstick cooking
spray
2 cups packaged hash
brown potatoes or
fresh-grated potato

9 oz. small broccoli florets
(rinsed and drained, but
not dried—some water
droplets should cling to
the broccoli)

4 eggs

4 egg whites

16 oz. container mushrooms,
    rinsed and dried

¼ cup skim milk

¼ tsp. black pepper

- Preheat the oven to 400°F.
- Lightly spray a medium ovenproof skillet with cooking
  spray. Heat over medium heat. Remove from the heat.
  Put the potatoes in the skillet. Lightly spray with
  cooking spray. Cook for 4–5 minutes, or until the
  potatoes are golden brown, stirring occasionally.
- Put the broccoli in a microwaveable bowl. Microwave,
  covered, on 100 percent power (high) for 4 to 5
  minutes, or until tender-crisp. Drain in a colander. Stir
  the broccoli into the potatoes.
- In a medium bowl, whisk together the egg whites and
  eggs. Whisk in the mushrooms, milk, and pepper. Pour
  the mixture over the potatoes and broccoli, stirring well.
- Bake for 15–18 minutes, or until the eggs are set (it
  shouldn't move much when the frittata is gently shaken).
- Let cool for at least 10 minutes, then cut into 2–4
  equal slices.

2 servings

SPICY FISH TACOS

½ cup salsa or pico de gallo

1 lime, juiced

1 tbsp. chopped fresh
    cilantro

1 tsp. chili powder

Salt and pepper, to taste

1 ¼ lbs. firm white fish
    such as tilapia or halibut

½ cup Greek plain yogurt
1 tbsp. hot sauce

Eight 6-inch corn tortillas
(warmed)

- In a medium bowl, whisk together the salsa, lime juice, cilantro, chili powder, salt, and pepper. Set aside.
- Coat a large sauté pan with cooking spray. Sauté fish over medium heat for 2 minutes on each side. Pour salsa mixture over fish and sauté an additional 3 minutes.
- Remove the fish from the pan and flake with a fork, mixing in the salsa mixture.
- In a small bowl, combine the yogurt and hot sauce. Evenly divide the fish among 8 tortillas and top each with a dollop of the yogurt sauce.

Makes 8 tacos, serving is 3 tacos

BAKED TERIYAKI CHICKEN

½ tbsp. cornstarch
½ tbsp. cold water
¼ cup Splenda granulated sweetener
¼ cup lower-sodium soy sauce

2 tbsp. apple cider vinegar
1 clove garlic, minced
½ tsp. ground ginger
¼ tsp. black pepper
1 ½ lbs. boneless, skinless chicken breasts

- Preheat oven to 425°F. Spray a 9- by 13-inch baking dish with cooking spray.
- In a saucepan, whisk together cornstarch and cold water until smooth. Whisk in Splenda sweetener, soy sauce, vinegar, garlic, ginger, and pepper. Bring to a

simmer over low heat and cook, stirring frequently, until sauce thickens and bubbles.

- Place chicken in prepared baking dish and brush with teriyaki sauce. Turn chicken over, and brush again.
- Bake for 15 minutes. Turn chicken and bake until chicken is no longer pink and juices run clear when pierced with the tip of a paring knife (20–30 minutes total baking time, depending on size). Brush with sauce every 10 minutes during baking.
- If you choose not to use Splenda, substitute 2 tbsp. table sugar for the whole recipe.

6 servings

5-INGREDIENT CHICKEN TORTILLA SOUP

4 cups chicken stock
1 rotisserie chicken, shredded
1 (19 oz.) can red enchilada sauce
1 (14 oz.) can fire-roasted tomatoes, diced
1 (14 oz.) can creamed or sweet corn
One 6-to-8-inch flour tortilla (or crushed tortilla chips)
1 tsp. olive oil

- Cut the tortilla into thin strips. Place in a frying pan with oil and cook until crispy.
- Place all ingredients into a large soup pot and bring to a boil.
- Simmer for 15 minutes.
- Ladle soup into bowls and serve with your favorite fixings.

4 servings

BBQ CHICKEN PIZZA

Nonstick cooking spray
½ lb. boneless, skinless
  chicken breast
¼ tsp. salt
¼ tsp. black pepper
¼ cup sugar-free apricot
  preserves
¼ cup barbeque sauce
½ tsp. hot sauce

12-inch prepackaged
  whole wheat pizza crust
1 cup shredded carrots
½ medium red onion,
  thinly sliced
½ cup reduced-fat
  shredded Italian-style
  cheese
½ tsp. dried oregano

- Preheat the oven to 375°F. Spray a baking sheet with cooking spray.
- Season the chicken with salt and pepper on both sides.
- Place the chicken on the prepared baking sheet and bake for 25 minutes or until the juices run clear. Remove the chicken from the oven and chop into half-inch pieces.
- In a small saucepan, combine the sugar-free apricot preserves, barbeque sauce, and hot sauce. Bring to a boil.
- Spoon the sauce over the pizza crust. Top the crust with cooked chicken, carrot, sliced onion, and cheese. Sprinkle the cheese with the dried oregano.
- Bake the pizza for 20–25 minutes or until the cheese is melted and bubbly.

4 servings (2 slices a serving)

ALASKAN SALMON WITH ORANGE WATERCRESS

4 Alaskan salmon filets (4–6 oz. each, frozen or fresh)

¼ cup avocado oil, divided

Bunches (about 3 cups watercress, roughly chopped)

3 tbsp. cucumber(s), finely chopped

2 oranges (peeled and segmented, membrane removed)

1 tsp. white wine vinegar

1 pinch salt and pepper, to taste

2 cups mixed greens

½ avocado, pitted, peeled, and sliced

¼ cup walnuts

2 tbsp. apple cider vinegar

- Rinse any ice glaze from Alaskan salmon under cold water; pat dry with paper towel. Heat skillet over medium-high heat and brush both sides of fish using 3 tablespoons of avocado oil. Cook salmon, uncovered, about 4 minutes, until browned.
- Turn salmon over and season lightly with salt and pepper. Cook an additional 6–8 minutes for frozen, or 3–4 minutes for fresh/thawed, just until fish is opaque throughout.
- Meanwhile, in a medium bowl, combine watercress, cucumber, and orange segments. Season with a few drops of white wine vinegar, remaining avocado oil, and salt and pepper, to taste.
- Plate mixed greens next to salmon and top with avocado, walnuts, and apple cider vinaigrette.

8 servings

BEEF FAJITAS

2 tsp. canola oil
2 cups sliced onion
2 cups sliced bell peppers
20 oz. cooked sliced steak

¼ tsp. salt
4 (8-inch) whole wheat
 flour tortillas

- Heat the oil in a large nonstick skillet over medium-high heat. Add the onion and bell pepper. Sauté for 5 minutes. Add the cooked sliced steak and sauté for 2–3 minutes to warm. Sprinkle with salt.
- Wrap the tortillas in damp paper towels and microwave on high for 1 minute.
- Place each tortilla on a plate. Divide the steak, onions, and peppers among the 4 tortillas. Wrap and serve. These fajitas go well with a green salad.

4 servings

WEEK FOUR AVERAGE NUTRITIONAL BREAKDOWN	
37% CARBS, 24% PROTEIN, 33% FAT	
Calories: 1,507	Fat: 54g
Carbohydrates: 140g	Fiber: 29g
Protein: 90g	Added sugar: 3g

WEEK ONE				
	BREAKFAST	LUNCH	SNACK	DINNER	TOTALS

	BREAKFAST	LUNCH	SNACK	DINNER	TOTALS
MONDAY	Calories: 352 Carbs: 46g Protein: 12g Fat: 1g Fiber: 12g Added sugar: 0g	Calories: 369 Carbs: 48g Protein: 26g Fat: 10g Fiber: 11g Added sugar: 0g	Calories: 242 Carbs: 11g Protein: 12g Fat: 8g Fiber: 3g Added sugar: 0g	Calories: 570 Carbs: 60g Protein: 29g Fat: 12g Fiber: 7g Added sugar: 4g	Calories: 1,533 Carbs: 165g Protein: 79g Fat: 31g Fiber: 33g Added sugar: 4g
TUESDAY	Calories: 310 Carbs: 42g Protein: 14g Fat: 10g Fiber: 4g Added sugar: 0g	Calories: 375 Carbs: 45g Protein: 16g Fat: 3.4g Fiber: 11.4g Added sugar: 0g	Calories: 268 Carbs: 33g Protein: 7g Fat: 14g Fiber: 7g Added sugar: 0g	Calories: 403 Carbs: 46g Protein: 26g Fat: 8.6g Fiber: 4.3g Added sugar: 2g	Calories: 1,356 Carbs: 166g Protein: 63g Fat: 36g Fiber: 26g Added sugar: 2g
WEDNESDAY	Calories: 350 Carbs: 45g Protein: 8g Fat: 0g Fiber: 9g Added sugar: 0g	Calories: 364 Carbs: 36g Protein: 25g Fat: 13g Fiber: 2.3g Added sugar: 0g	Calories: 234 Carbs: 39g Protein: 10g Fat: 5g Fiber: 5g Added sugar: 0g	Calories: 330 Carbs: 50g Protein: 18.6g Fat: 8g Fiber: 4g Added sugar: 0g	Calories: 1,278 Carbs: 170g Protein: 62g Fat: 26g Fiber: 20g Added sugar: 0g
THURSDAY	Calories: 522 Carbs: 58g Protein: 15g Fat: 10g Fiber: 13g Added sugar: 0g	Calories: 388 Carbs: 34g Protein: 10g Fat: 16g Fiber: 6g Added sugar: 0g	Calories: 240 Carbs: 22g Protein: 29g Fat: 5g Fiber: 3g Added sugar: 0g	Calories: 388 Carbs: 52g Protein: 17g Fat: 15g Fiber: 6.3g Added sugar: 0g	Calories: 1,538 Carbs: 166g Protein: 71g Fat: 46g Fiber: 33g Added sugar: 0g
FRIDAY	Calories: 414 Carbs: 39g Protein: 22g Fat: 23g Fiber: 5g Added sugar: 0g	Calories: 278 Carbs: 25g Protein: 31g Fat: 6g Fiber: 8g Added sugar: 0g	Calories: 313 Carbs: 39g Protein: 9g Fat: 15g Fiber: 5g Added sugar: 2g	Calories: 489 Carbs: 47g Protein: 28g Fat: 14g Fiber: 11g Added sugar: 0g	Calories: 1,494 Carbs: 177g Protein: 90g Fat: 60g Fiber: 29g Added sugar: 2g
SATURDAY	Calories: 361 Carbs: 48g Protein: 16g Fat: 11g Fiber: 7g Added sugar: 0g	Calories: 350 Carbs: 15g Protein: 16g Fat: 25g Fiber: 7g Added sugar: 0g	Calories: 350 Carbs: 38g Protein: 7g Fat: 6g Fiber: 3g Added sugar: 0g	Calories: 487 Carbs: 60g Protein: 24.2g Fat: 16g Fiber: 8g Added sugar: 0g	Calories: 1,548 Carbs:161g Protein: 63g Fat: 58g Fiber: 25g Added sugar: 0g
SUNDAY	Calories: 399 Carbs: 45g Protein: 24g Fat: 13g Fiber: 15g Added sugar: 0g	Calories: 408 Carbs: 20g Protein: 26g Fat: 25g Fiber: 8g Added sugar: 0g	Calories: 291 Carbs: 30g Protein: 3g Fat: 3g Fiber: 5g Added sugar: 0g	Calories: 336 Carbs: 45g Protein: 24g Fat: 12g Fiber: 12g Added sugar: 3g	Calories: 1,434 Carbs: 141g Protein: 77g Fat: 53g Fiber: 40g Added sugar: 3g

	BREAKFAST	LUNCH	SNACK	DINNER	TOTALS
WEEK TWO					
MONDAY	Calories: 307 Carbs: 27g Protein: 12g Fat: 14g Fiber: 9g Added sugar: 0g	Calories: 304 Carbs: 21g Protein: 22g Fat: 16g Fiber: 12g Added sugar: 0g	Calories: 245 Carbs: 23g Protein: 12g Fat: 10g Fiber: 3g Added sugar: 0g	Calories: 401 Carbs: 39g Protein: 35g Fat: 14g Fiber: 10g Added sugar: 0g	Calories: 1,257 Carbs: 110g Protein: 81g Fat: 44g Fiber: 34g Added sugar: 0g
TUESDAY	Calories: 249 Carbs: 23g Protein: 20g Fat: 10g Fiber: 6g Added sugar: 0g	Calories: 432 Carbs: 33g Protein: 13g Fat: 32g Fiber: 13g Added sugar: 0g	Calories: 278 Carbs: 25g Protein: 15g Fat: 1g Fiber: 9g Added sugar: 0g	Calories: 602 Carbs: 60g Protein: 13g Fat: 30g Fiber: 15g Added sugar: 0g	Calories: 1,561 Carbs: 141g Protein: 61g Fat: 73g Fiber: 43g Added sugar: 0g
WEDNESDAY	Calories: 350 Carbs: 45g Protein: 10g Fat: 15g Fiber: 9g Added sugar: 3g	Calories: 379 Carbs: 28g Protein: 33g Fat: 15g Fiber: 9g Added sugar: 0g	Calories: 296 Carbs: 38g Protein: 6g Fat: 15g Fiber: 5g Added sugar: 0g	Calories: 369 Carbs: 38g Protein: 18g Fat: 14g Fiber: 6g Added sugar: 0g	Calories: 1,394 Carbs: 149g Protein: 67g Fat: 59g Fiber: 28g Added sugar: 3g
THURSDAY	Calories: 391 Carbs: 52g Protein: 21g Fat: 12g Fiber: 5g Added sugar: 1g	Calories: 425 Carbs: 60g Protein: 25g Fat: 27g Fiber: 7g Added sugar: 0g	Calories: 263 Carbs: 14g Protein: 15g Fat: 18g Fiber: 5.5g Added sugar: 0g	Calories: 434 Carbs: 55g Protein: 31g Fat: 10g Fiber: 4g Added sugar: 0g	Calories: 1,513 Carbs: 181g Protein: 92g Fat: 67g Fiber: 28g Added sugar: 1g
FRIDAY	Calories: 361 Carbs: 44g Protein: 21g Fat: 11g Fiber: 7g Added sugar: 0g	Calories: 380 Carbs: 30g Protein: 29g Fat: 16g Fiber: 8g Added sugar: 0g	Calories: 351 Carbs: 41g Protein: 10g Fat: 19g Fiber: 9g Added sugar: 0g	Calories: 508 Carbs: 28g Protein: 40g Fat: 22g Fiber: 6g Added sugar: 0g	Calories: 1,600 Carbs: 143g Protein: 100g Fat: 68g Fiber: 30g Added sugar: 0g
SATURDAY	Calories: 275 Carbs: 20g Protein: 11g Fat: 3g Fiber: 4g Added sugar: 5g	Calories: 220 Carbs: 21g Protein: 25g Fat: 9g Fiber: 14g Added sugar: 0g	Calories: 265 Carbs: 24g Protein: 10g Fat: 16g Fiber: 10g Added sugar: 0g	Calories: 609 Carbs: 45g Protein: 36g Fat: 31g Fiber: 13g Added sugar: 0g	Calories: 1,369 Carbs: 110g Protein: 82g Fat: 59g Fiber: 41g Added sugar: 5g
SUNDAY	Calories: 300 Carbs: 19g Protein: 17g Fat: 13g Fiber: 4g Added sugar: 0g	Calories: 477 Carbs: 46g Protein: 34g Fat: 17g Fiber: 15g Added sugar: 0g	Calories: 265 Carbs: 51g Protein: 10g Fat: 3g Fiber: 10g Added sugar: 0g	Calories: 530 Carbs: 25g Protein: 24g Fat: 35g Fiber: 6g Added sugar: 0g	Calories: 1,572 Carbs: 141g Protein: 85g Fat: 68g Fiber: 35g Added sugar: 0g

WEEK THREE				
	BREAKFAST	LUNCH	SNACK	DINNER	TOTALS
MONDAY	Calories: 418 Carbs: 30g Protein: 12g Fat: 13g Fiber: 4g Added sugar: 2g	Calories: 428 Carbs: 27g Protein: 28g Fat: 18g Fiber: 6g Added sugar: 0g	Calories: 273 Carbs: 51g Protein: 19g Fat: 1g Fiber: 6g Added sugar: 0g	Calories: 417 Carbs: 40g Protein: 21g Fat: 10g Fiber: 6g Added sugar: 5g	Calories: 1,536 Carbs: 148g Protein: 80g Fat: 42g Fiber: 22g Added sugar: 5g
TUESDAY	Calories: 245 Carbs: 23g Protein: 13g Fat: 12g Fiber: 4g Added sugar: 0g	Calories: 299 Carbs: 35g Protein: 7g Fat: 11g Fiber: 4g Added sugar: 0g	Calories: 285 Carbs: 20g Protein: 14g Fat: 15g Fiber: 7g Added sugar: 0g	Calories: 442 Carbs: 50g Protein: 19g Fat: 6g Fiber: 10g Added sugar: 0g	Calories: 1,271 Carbs: 128g Protein: 53g Fat: 53g Fiber: 25g Added sugar: 0g
WEDNESDAY	Calories: 317 Carbs: 60g Protein: 13g Fat: 4g Fiber: 6g Added sugar: 3g	Calories: 335 Carbs: 50g Protein: 12g Fat: 10g Fiber: 8g Added sugar: 0g	Calories: 299 Carbs: 35g Protein: 30g Fat: 6g Fiber: 11g Added sugar: 0g	Calories: 520 Carbs: 50g Protein: 29g Fat: 16g Fiber: 7g Added sugar: 0g	Calories: 1,471 Carbs: 195g Protein: 84g Fat: 36g Fiber: 32g Added sugar: 3g
THURSDAY	Calories: 303 Carbs: 44g Protein: 15g Fat: 10g Fiber: 4g Added sugar: 10g	Calories: 625 Carbs: 40g Protein: 32g Fat: 40g Fiber: 15g Added sugar: 0g	Calories: 304 Carbs: 28g Protein: 30g Fat: 6g Fiber: 6g Added sugar: 0g	Calories: 400 Carbs: 40g Protein: 20g Fat: 12g Fiber: 7g Added sugar: 0g	Calories: 1,632 Carbs: 152g Protein: 97g Fat: 68g Fiber: 32g Added sugar: 10g
FRIDAY	Calories: 310 Carbs: 33g Protein: 6g Fat: 19g Fiber: 6g Added sugar: 2g	Calories: 317 Carbs: 47g Protein: 13g Fat: 8g Fiber: 5g Added sugar: 0g	Calories: 251 Carbs: 28g Protein: 20g Fat: 7g Fiber: 4g Added sugar: 0g	Calories: 500 Carbs: 36g Protein: 26g Fat: 10g Fiber: 10g Added sugar: 0g	Calories: 1,378 Carbs: 144g Protein: 65g Fat: 44g Fiber: 25g Added sugar: 2g
SATURDAY	Calories: 348 Carbs: 27g Protein: 15g Fat: 21g Fiber: 8g Added sugar: 0g	Calories: 478 Carbs: 56g Protein: 10g Fat: 26g Fiber: 9g Added sugar: 0g	Calories: 295 Carbs: 25g Protein: 12g Fat: 18g Fiber: 14g Added sugar: 0g	Calories: 350 Carbs: 45g Protein: 14g Fat: 6g Fiber: 11g Added sugar: 0g	Calories: 1,471 Carbs: 153g Protein: 51g Fat: 71g Fiber: 42g Added sugar: 0g
SUNDAY	Calories: 340 Carbs: 20g Protein: 31g Fat: 19g Fiber: 4g Added sugar: 0g	Calories: 415 Carbs: 58g Protein: 30g Fat: 7g Fiber: 14g Added sugar: 0g	Calories: 348 Carbs: 20g Protein: 19g Fat: 21g Fiber: 6g Added sugar: 0g	Calories: 400 Carbs: 30g Protein: 29g Fat: 9g Fiber: 6g Added sugar: 0g	Calories: 1,503 Carbs: 128g Protein: 109g Fat: 56g Fiber: 30g Added sugar: 0g

	BREAKFAST	LUNCH	SNACK	DINNER	TOTALS
WEEK FOUR					
MONDAY	Calories: 300 Carbs: 15g Protein: 15g Fat: 17g Fiber: 2g Added sugar: 0g	Calories: 489 Carbs: 46g Protein: 40g Fat: 15g Fiber: 5g Added sugar: 0g	Calories: 359 Carbs: 18g Protein: 14g Fat: 28g Fiber: 9g Added sugar: 0g	Calories: 450 Carbs: 45g Protein: 45g Fat: 8g Fiber: 9g Added sugar: 0g	Calories: 1,598 Carbs: 124g Protein: 114g Fat: 68g Fiber: 25g Added sugar: 0g
TUESDAY	Calories: 170 Carbs: 20g Protein: 14g Fat: 4.5g Fiber: 3g Added sugar: 0g	Calories: 394 Carbs: 20g Protein: 15g Fat: 30g Fiber: 6g Added sugar: 0g	Calories: 405 Carbs: 28g Protein: 40g Fat: 12g Fiber: 4g Added sugar: 0g	Calories: 604 Carbs: 60g Protein: 25g Fat: 28g Fiber: 12g Added sugar: 0g	Calories: 1,573 Carbs: 128g Protein: 94g Fat: 75g Fiber: 25g Added sugar: 0g
WEDNESDAY	Calories: 287 Carbs: 28g Protein: 23g Fat: 10g Fiber: 5g Added sugar: 0g	Calories: 611 Carbs: 60g Protein: 24g Fat: 27g Fiber: 13g Added sugar: 0g	Calories: 365 Carbs: 52g Protein: 7g Fat: 15g Fiber: 10g Added sugar: 0g	Calories: 420 Carbs: 25g Protein: 30g Fat: 4g Fiber: 10g Added sugar: 1g	Calories: 1,683 Carbs: 165g Protein: 84g Fat: 56g Fiber: 38g Added sugar: 1g
THURSDAY	Calories: 304 Carbs: 35g Protein: 11g Fat: 4g Fiber: 5g Added sugar: 4g	Calories: 200 Carbs: 30g Protein: 10g Fat: 2g Fiber: 6g Added sugar: 0g	Calories: 282 Carbs: 10g Protein: 16g Fat: 12g Fiber: 5g Added sugar: 0g	Calories: 425 Carbs: 45g Protein: 20g Fat: 7g Fiber: 9g Added sugar: 0g	Calories: 1,211 Carbs: 120g Protein: 67g Fat: 25g Fiber: 25g Added sugar: 4g
FRIDAY	Calories: 425 Carbs: 47g Protein: 19g Fat: 21g Fiber: 7g Added sugar: 0g	Calories: 480 Carbs: 25g Protein: 40g Fat: 21g Fiber: 5g Added sugar: 0g	Calories: 332 Carbs: 45g Protein: 17g Fat: 12g Fiber: 8g Added sugar: 10g	Calories: 320 Carbs: 46g Protein: 22g Fat: 7g Fiber: 12g Added sugar: 4g	Calories: 1,557 Carbs: 163g Protein: 98g Fat: 61g Fiber: 32g Added sugar: 14g
SATURDAY	Calories: 240 Carbs: 37g Protein: 12g Fat: 5g Fiber: 6g Added sugar: 0g	Calories: 256 Carbs: 13g Protein: 19g Fat: 14g Fiber: 4g Added sugar: 0g	Calories: 500 Carbs: 43g Protein: 7g Fat: 14g Fiber: 8g Added sugar: 0g	Calories: 482 Carbs: 40g Protein: 40g Fat: 19g Fiber: 8g Added sugar: 0g	Calories: 1,478 Carbs: 133g Protein: 78g Fat: 52g Fiber: 26g Added sugar: 0g
SUNDAY	Calories: 340 Carbs: 38g Protein: 25g Fat: 9g Fiber: 7g Added sugar: 0g	Calories: 335 Carbs: 60g Protein: 11g Fat: 4g Fiber: 9g Added sugar: 0g	Calories: 307 Carbs: 25g Protein: 20g Fat: 14g Fiber: 5g Added sugar: 0g	Calories: 470 Carbs: 35g Protein: 39g Fat: 16g Fiber: 9g Added sugar: 0g	Calories: 1,452 Carbs: 150g Protein: 99g Fat: 45g Fiber: 30g Added sugar: 0g

CHAPTER SIX

How to Harness the Power of Exercise

TRUE OR FALSE?

1. Fifteen minutes of exercise a day is enough to get healthy.
2. Cardio is much more important than lifting weights.
3. Vigorous exercise lowers your blood sugar.
4. Building muscle replaces fat.
5. Doing chores around the house counts as "exercise."

(Answers at end of chapter)

DO YOU NEED ME TO tell you to exercise? Probably not. You know you should be exercising—we all know it, but we're simply not getting up off the couch to do it (or if we are, it's just barely—"does walking to the refrigerator count?"). Let's face it—exercise just doesn't feel pressing. Our body doesn't set off a "must exercise!" alarm like it does for hunger or sleep deprivation, so it's easy to dismiss exercise as simply a "nice to have." We can tell ourselves that it's something we only need to do if we really want to look and feel better; but if we're happy enough with how our body is then it's not worth the effort. We don't think of exercise as something we need to do to survive. After all, if it were that important, wouldn't your body sound an alarm telling you to do it?

Your high blood sugar *is* that alarm. Sadly, we often don't hear it—or we ignore it, or "snooze" it.

Sure, there are some people who enjoy getting up at 5:00 a.m. to head to the gym or go on a ten-mile run and feel invigorated. But many of us simply don't really understand what we need to do or can't seem to make a commitment to do it. Is exercise worth the time?

If you want to reverse diabetes or delay some of the health consequences, you must incorporate daily exercise and physical activity into your life. There's simply no getting around it. The good news is it doesn't have to be as hard as you may think, and the benefits are well worth your time. One of my goals in this book is to help you create a love affair with exercise. I don't want you to just like it—I want you to love it! You are probably thinking you have tried exercise in the past with limited success. We have all been there. We start off pretty good but then "life happens," and we just can't seem to fit exercise in. But it's important to let go of your past efforts and allow yourself to have a fresh start. We consider "exercise" expendable or a low priority—when, in fact, we *need* to exercise to take control of our diabetes risk. Part of the solution is helping you to change how you think about it—and that starts with getting a clear understanding of just how important exercise really is. We often say "we need to go to work." How do we modify that to also say "we need to go work out"?

Cultivate the mindset that you are not going to let barriers prevent you from getting active. I've heard all the excuses from "I need to get in shape before I can start exercising" to "I don't want to get injured." I myself have used many of these excuses. When you don't exercise, you are missing out on reducing your risk of diabetes and its complications.

You might not realize the specific and targeted effect exercise has on prediabetes and diabetes. It's one of the best strategies to reverse and prevent complications of your high blood sugar.

How so? It does so in a couple of different ways.

First, exercise lowers your blood sugar and makes you more insulin sensitive, which slashes your odds of developing prediabetes. It does that by amping up the ability of your muscles to soak up and dispose of the glucose in your bloodstream— turning your muscles, quite simply, into metabolic sponges. Studies show that while you are exercising, the amount of glucose taken up by your muscles increases fivefold, and this elevation in glucose uptake can last up to forty-eight hours. That makes it a lot easier for insulin, which escorts glucose into your cells, to do its job. Numerous studies have demonstrated that people with prediabetes who were assigned to engage in regular exercise slashed their risk of progressing to diabetes by 46 percent, which was even better than the group that was assigned to follow a healthy diet without engaging in regular exercise (that group reduced their risk of diabetes by 31 percent).

Secondly, it helps your liver decrease the amount of glucose it needs to produce for your energy needs. It's probably because muscles can use glucose without insulin when you are exercising. This is a powerful effect! It helps your blood glucose levels go down. Just as exercise makes your muscles grow, it also makes the beta cells in your pancreas grow, improving how you make insulin.

The reason exercise has to be a part of your lifestyle and not just something you do to reach a certain goal is because these benefits are reversible—meaning when you stop routinely exercising, the benefits go away. That's why exercise needs to be incorporated into how you live. Just as you need to focus on what you eat, you need to focus on your activity. Please don't have the attitude that you will exercise for a few weeks or a couple months to reach a weight-loss goal. I urge you to avoid the classic "lose twenty pounds in twenty days" mentality. In more than twenty-five years of practice, I've never seen those approaches work long term—because they are designed for the short term! In these circumstances, patients typically regain that weight, and more. It can be extremely frustrating and demoralizing. The key to reversing diabetes or preventing or delaying side effects through exercise is to think both short and long term, incorporating exercise into your lifestyle most days of the week.

You should also think about what the effects of *not* exercising will be. Because you're not getting the benefits of exercise, you're potentially making your condition worse—reducing your chances of reversal or at least preventing complications.

Beyond diabetes control, exercise has a wide range of other health benefits. We tend to think that the primary benefit is weight loss and, indeed, by burning more calories, you will likely lose weight, get rid of fat, and build muscle. But don't think exercise is just about weight loss. There are life-changing benefits far beyond losing some pounds. And for those that are normal weight, you still get lots of benefits.

Here are just a few:

- Lowers your bad cholesterol and increases your good cholesterol.
- Strengthens your bones, delaying or preventing osteoporosis.
- Increases muscle endurance, maintains muscle mass, and promotes joint flexibility.

- Releases endorphins, helping to reduce anxiety and depression.
- Improves the quality of your sleep, which we now know impacts both the length and quality of our lives.
- Makes your blood vessels more flexible, improves blood flow and circulation, helping to control your blood pressure. It improves your heart function and decreases risk of heart attack and strokes.
- Enhances your metabolism.
- Slows the aging process.

Have I convinced you? Instead of taking a pill or a shot, focus on exercise as part of your treatment plan to take control of your diabetes risk. You won't find a pill that has all these benefits—and very few side effects!

How Much Is Enough?

Now is a good time to review what I mean by "exercise." Patients often tell me they are always "running errands" or "active around the house" or "walking around at work." Does that count? It depends.

We tend to use the words *exercise* and *physical activity* interchangeably, but they do have subtle differences. Exercise is a planned and structured session of activity carried out to improve or maintain one or more aspects of fitness. Physical activity is any movement of the body. It can be anything from running to standing up from a chair. All forms of exercise are physical activity, but all physical activity is not exercise.

For you to achieve benefits to reduce your elevated blood sugar, I want you to think "exercise." It's not just words—it's a mindset. Research demonstrates that regular exercise may prevent or delay type 2 diabetes and give health benefits to people with type 1.

The American Diabetes Association currently recommends 150 minutes per week of moderate-intensity physical activity. That sounds like a lot, doesn't it? When you break it down, that's less than thirty minutes a day. When you realize that exercise can treat your diabetes as effectively as some medicines, exercise is well worth your time. In fact, you need to be doing it. What's particularly exciting is that "more may be better." By that, I mean the benefits are proportional to exercise volume—meaning the more you do, the more exercise benefits the management of your diabetes.

Ideally, exercise should be fun—that way, you will be more likely to stick with it. But exercise does require effort, and sometimes it will be work. And you will always have excuses: you won't feel like doing it; you forgot your gym clothes; you don't want to get up early; you don't want to get sweaty; you don't know what to do. We all have felt this way at times. But we can't let those thoughts have the final say. Remember, exercise can be as powerful as prescription medicines. And you don't skip taking your prescriptions, right?

Unfortunately, only about 25 percent of people with diabetes follow the ADA's exercise recommendations. That's only one in four. I wish my doctor colleagues would consider writing an actual exercise prescription detailing what you need to do daily. It would convey how important it is to engage in exercise. I recognize that some days you realistically just cannot do it. And you don't have to exercise every day of the week to reap the benefits. But once or twice a week is not enough. I always tell patients not to let more than two days elapse between exercise sessions. Once you start letting days pass in between sessions, it becomes harder and harder to maintain a routine. And you also start to lose the benefits, so making it a routine is key.

One of the beauties of exercise is there's so much variety. I don't like to get too bogged down in terms and definitions. There's no need to make it overly complicated. When it comes to different types of exercise, I always tell people to divide it into aerobic, resistance, and flexibility, incorporating all of them into your lifestyle.

Types of Exercise

TYPES OF EXERCISE

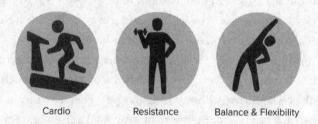

Cardio   Resistance   Balance & Flexibility

Aerobic exercise (sometimes referred to as "cardio") involves repeated and continuous movement of large muscle groups. For those lovers of words, aerobic means "with oxygen." Aerobic exercise causes your blood to deliver oxygen to those muscles that are working. Think walking, jogging, bicycling, swimming, skiing, dancing, and that Zumba class your friend is trying to take you to!

The reason aerobic exercise is so important in helping to manage prediabetes or diabetes is that it dramatically increases the uptake of glucose by your muscles—nearly five times your resting rate. It also enhances the work of insulin, so you don't need as much. These benefits often last for several hours after you finish exercise. You get benefits for longer than the time you spend exercising. That should be exciting to hear.

I bet many of you do cardio. Too often, however, people rely only on cardio and that's not enough—you aren't exercising hard enough to get the specific benefits you're aiming for. For instance, let's talk about step-counting. I have a few friends—and family members—that are very focused on their daily step count. And some are always challenging. Walking is a great way to get healthy. But you also need to experience exertion—sometimes, you might need to "power walk." I have many patients who walk over ten thousand steps a day but still are overweight with a low fitness level. Exercise requires effort to reap the rewards. To get maximum benefit, you need to make sure you elevate your heart rate and get your breathing up. That's where a smartwatch can come in handy.

Another type of exercise is anaerobic exercise. Anaerobic means "without oxygen," so these types of physical activities break down glucose without using oxygen. They're typically exercises that are briefer but more intense than aerobic exercises. They include activities like resistance training (such as weight-lifting), sprinting, and high-intensity interval training. Whereas aerobic helps with your heart, anerobic helps with your muscle strength.

I don't want you to think that resistance training means you need to buy equipment or sign up for a gym membership and start pumping iron. A lot of resistance training can be done with the weight of your own body. My favorite is the push-up—there are very few excuses that will prevent you from doing push-ups. You don't need any special equipment or a big space. They can be done almost anytime, anywhere. And they're effective: data shows that men who can do forty push-ups live longer than men who can do ten or fewer.

What about stretching? Should you stretch before or after exercise? Most recent data suggests that stretching before working out does not prevent injury; instead, warm up with a few repetitions of your exercises at low intensity. After a workout, stretching doesn't seem to prevent soreness as much as many people think. Instead of deciding whether you do it before or after, make stretching its own routine. It does increase the range of motion of your joints, but it doesn't affect glycemic control. Its value is different from exercise. I recommend stretching—it's good for your body overall and can improve the quality of your cardio and resistance training sessions—but you can't count it as your exercise program. It won't reduce your risk of prediabetes or diabetes.

I remind people that as we get older it is important to incorporate exercises that promote flexibility and balance. Flexibility involves range of motion around joints. Balance focuses on how you walk. Both are critically important in preventing injury and disability. As we age our muscles become tighter, scarred, and shorter and our nerves aren't as quick to respond to their needs. Working on stretching and balance helps keep us young and reduces the risk of falls and injuries.

Here's a tip: tai chi incorporates it all—flexibility, balance, and resistance!

Some Is Better Than None, Right?

As I mentioned, exercising for 150 minutes a week is the goal I want you to reach, ideally averaging 30 minutes 5 days a week. I recognize that it will take some time for many of you to get to that point. And some of you will feel that even twenty or thirty minutes just isn't doable most days—so you may wonder if some is better than none, right? Honestly, it's a bit more complicated. I'd be giving you bad information if I let you think that you can just do ten minutes a couple times a week.

Just as medicines have a dose, so, too, does exercise. And just as you need to take the required dose of medicine for it to have an effect, so, too, with exercise. If you exercise a little bit, but less than the recommended time and intensity, you will not get the benefits that your body needs (and so, you're really not making the best use of your time). Your dose of exercise really needs to be *at least* twenty to thirty minutes, four to five days a week. And I want you to exert yourself for much of this time. You need to get your heart rate into the moderate-intensity zone. (For moderate intensity physical activity, the target heart rate should be *50 to 70* percent of their maximum heart rate. The maximum rate is based on a person's age. An estimate of a person's maximum heart rate can be calculated as 220 beats per minute [bpm] minus your age.) You can use your smartphone or other devices to monitor your heart rate. Or you can go low tech and estimate your exercise intensity with the simple talk test. To perform the talk test, see if you can talk or sing while performing the activity. If you're doing a moderate exercise, you should be able to talk, but not sing. If you're doing a vigorous exercise, you shouldn't be able to say more than a few words. There's also the "perceived exertion" scale where basically intensity is determined by how you feel your heart rate and breathing. This can be good early on when you are starting an exercise program—listen to your body and learn how it responds.

Don't get me wrong: it's okay to *start* slowly and build up to 150 minutes a week over time. It may take you several months.

I just don't want you to do ten minutes of exercise a few times a week and think that is sufficient to reverse prediabetes or blunt the effects of diabetes—because it won't.

What Do I Need to Do?

Armed with this information, you might be wondering: Okay, so precisely what *type* of exercise should I do for treating or reversing diabetes? Everyone is going to be a little different based on their abilities, their health, age, and weight. For instance, you may be limited in what you can do as a result of age, underlying health issues, injuries, or skill level—but wherever you are, the most important thing is to *start*. You may need to begin by walking a few times a week at a moderate pace, and then work your way up to more challenging activities—that certainly beats sitting on the couch. But generally speaking, the more vigorous the exercise, the better. And, believe it or not, having physical limitations doesn't mean you can't get your heart pumping—you can work up a sweat even while you're sitting down with "chair aerobics" programs (a quick Google search will pull up lots of examples)!

Once you get started, look for ways to include different types of exercise in your routines. Research tells us that having variety in your workouts can help to reduce diabetes risk. Remember the Diabetes Prevention Program I mentioned earlier in the book? It showed that people at high risk of developing diabetes could prevent or delay the disease through diet and exercise. People in the study improved their diets and were instructed to do at least 150 minutes of primarily aerobic exercise each week that was similar in intensity to brisk walking. In addition to walking, the participants were also encouraged to add physical activities like aerobic dance, bike riding, skating, and swimming. This lifestyle intervention—which was designed to help the participants lose at least 7 percent of their body weight—was very successful, leading to a 58 percent reduction in the overall rate of diabetes.

And in recent years, studies have found that resistance training offers many of the same benefits as aerobic exercise, including improvements in blood sugar control. One recent study looked at what happened when people with diabetes or prediabetes did a forty-five-minute session of resistance training on one day and moderate-intensity aerobic activity on another day. Both types of exercise produced at least a 30 percent reduction in the prevalence of high blood sugar episodes over the twenty-four hours after exercise. Other large studies have found that both resistance training and aerobic exercise improve insulin sensitivity and lower your hemoglobin HbA1c.

We've also learned the importance of muscle strength in reducing diabetes risk. We did so by studying avid runners. Researchers found that runners who avoid strength training can experience significant muscle loss—known as sarcopenia—in their upper bodies despite having muscular legs. You want to avoid this—and not just for aesthetic reasons. Studies have found that adults with relatively low levels of muscle compared to others their age have double the risk of developing diabetes. Muscle plays a critical role in your metabolic health because it is one of the primary tissues that clear glucose from your bloodstream. You don't have to become a bodybuilder. But having a decent amount of muscle leads to greater glucose disposal, which can delay the onset of diabetes. That's one reason it's important to do some form of strength training.

But don't think, "Well, maybe if I don't have time for a cardio workout, I should just lift weights." People who lift weights

without doing any running or other forms of endurance training can experience sharp declines in their cardiorespiratory
fitness. Think of strength training as something that helps you
build a metabolic coat of armor: the lean muscle you'll add to
your frame will improve your blood sugar control and protect
you against falls, injuries, and weight gain as you get older.
Aerobic training will have a similar impact on your blood sugar
while also enhancing your cardiovascular health. Each is powerful on their own, but the sum is greater than its parts. Try not
to neglect either one.

Think You Have No Time to Exercise? What About a Few Minutes?

For some people, 150 minutes a week is going to be a real challenge sometimes. I get it—there are only so many hours in a day.
Lack of time is, after all, the number one reason people cite for
not exercising. There are some exceptions to the suggestion of
150 minutes weekly, but it requires different types and styles of
exercise. If you're pressed for time but don't want to miss out
on the benefits of exercise, you may want to consider high-
intensity interval training. Often referred to as HIIT and long
used by elite athletes, this type of workout involves doing extremely short bursts of vigorous exercise followed by very brief
periods of rest. In recent years, an explosion of research has
shown that high-intensity interval training might provide greater
metabolic benefits than other forms of exercise. And best of all,
it's quick and efficient. Thanks to HIIT, some people can get all
the benefits of regular exercise in a fraction of the time—minutes, in some cases—along with even sharper reductions in body
fat, inflammation, and blood sugar levels.

One of the best things about HIIT is that you can apply it to just about any form of exercise, including the simplest: walking. Several studies have looked at the impact of applying a HIIT protocol to walking—going at a vigorous pace for four minutes, then slowing to a low-intensity pace for three minutes and repeating this cycle four times. Researchers found that this strategy led to significantly greater improvements in cardiovascular health than the same amount of exercise performed at moderate intensity—and it only takes thirty minutes!

Want to make it even simpler? Consider this: some recent data showed that older adults with type 2 diabetes who did a "3 x 3" HIIT protocol for sixteen weeks—three minutes of fast walking followed by three minutes of slow walking and then repeated—had greater improvements in their body composition, aerobic fitness, and blood sugar control than a group that did the same amount of exercise at a moderate intensity. A comprehensive analysis found that in people with prediabetes, high-intensity interval training produced *double* the improvement in cardiorespiratory fitness compared to moderate-intensity exercise. Remember that poor cardiorespiratory fitness is a strong predictor of early death in people with diabetes.

The remarkable thing about high-intensity interval training is that more and more research shows that there are benefits seemingly no matter how low you go. One of my favorite forms of interval training is what's called "low-volume HIIT." This involves exercising at a hard intensity for one minute or less, resting for the same amount of time, and then repeating. If time is an issue for you, this approach might work for you because you can do this type of workout in less than twenty minutes and still see benefits. In a recent study, scientists recruited people with type 2 diabetes and instructed them do a short but intense "10-1" interval workout on a stationary bike: they cycled hard for one minute, rested for one minute, and repeated this cycle ten times, for a total workout time of just twenty minutes (ten minutes of actual exercise time plus ten minutes of rest). After two weeks of just three sessions of this per week—a total of one hour of working out per week—the participants saw significant reductions in their blood sugar levels and substantial improvements in their blood sugar responses to breakfast, lunch, and dinner.

Is ten minutes of exercise too much for you? Then how about a mere *two minutes of exercise?* A recent study tested the efficacy of a 4 x 30 second HIIT protocol that involved doing thirty seconds of exercise at a hard pace, followed by thirty seconds of rest, and repeating the cycle four times. That's a total workout time of only four minutes (two minutes of actual exercise and two minutes of rest). Amazingly, most of the participants in this study—middle-aged adults with diabetes—saw improvements in insulin resistance and reductions in their blood sugar levels after two weeks of doing just three sessions of this protocol. That's a total of only sixteen minutes a week of working out—less than the time it takes you to watch your favorite sitcom. Plenty of other studies have found that when it comes to optimizing your metabolic health and preventing prediabetes and other chronic conditions, high-intensity interval training always beats moderate-intensity exercise, regardless of the HIIT protocol you choose.

So why is this form of exercise so beneficial? Science shows us that the more vigorous the exercise, the more muscle fibers it recruits. As a result, your muscle glycogen levels are depleted at a faster rate, which leads to a greater increase in insulin sensitivity and, in turn, better blood sugar control. Because it is so demanding, high-intensity training burns more calories and glucose than moderate exercise. And over the long run, if you do it consistently, you'll achieve greater reductions in abdominal fat and larger improvements in muscle mass compared to low- or moderate-intensity training. All of this adds up to better metabolic health and a higher likelihood of living a long and healthy life. In one recent study, a team of Norwegian researchers recruited thousands of seniors and assigned them to one of three groups. The first group, which served as the control, was told to follow standard exercise guidelines. The second group was told to exercise moderately for about fifty minutes twice a week. And the third group did HIIT sessions twice a week, mostly jogging or cycling for four minutes on and then four minutes off several times per session. After five years, the researchers found that, on average, all the study participants tended to live longer than other people their age in the general population—demonstrating the value of exercise. But the HIIT group did the best of all. Compared to the control group and the moderate-intensity exercise group, they were less likely to die prematurely. They were also fitter and had a better quality of life than their peers. Need I say more?

HIIT is not for everyone. Some of you won't be able to sustain that level of exertion and some just won't like the style. If not done properly, there's a higher risk of injury. My point in including HIIT is to show you that there are lots of options nowadays to incorporate different types of exercise into your daily life.

Some Caveats

Although most people with prediabetes or even type 2 diabetes can safely engage in an exercise program, there are some special considerations—especially if your blood sugar is not under good control or if you are on insulin. It's also a good idea to speak with your doctor before you start.

- Drink plenty of fluids to prevent dehydration.
- Skip the gym if you aren't feeling well.
- Stop immediately if you develop dizziness, chest discomfort, or shortness of breath.
- If you are on insulin, you might want to check your blood sugar before you start. The ADA recommends that if it is below 100 mg/dl, you first eat a small snack. During exercise (especially if it is strenuous), low blood sugar is sometimes a concern.
- If your blood sugar is above 240 or 250, it may be too high, and you should probably wait to exercise. The concern would be that exercise might cause ketones to develop in your blood, which make it difficult for your brain, heart, and lungs to function properly. It's more likely in patients with type 1, rather than type 2, diabetes.
- Go slow. There's no race to get fit.

Risks of Exercise

If you begin to think of exercise as a "treatment" for diabetes, then just as with medications, there are risks and benefits. In general, the benefits of exercise far exceed any risks. The most common risks include exercise-related hypoglycemia (low blood sugar), dehydration, or a drop in blood pressure.

Exercise helps your body use glucose, but if you overdo exercise, it's possible your blood sugar might get too low. This tends to be more common in people using insulin or drugs that cause insulin to be released, or in those performing vigorous workouts or workouts that last more than sixty minutes. Signs to look out for include dizziness, excessive sweating, headache, shaking, nausea, or confusion. I always tell people that if you can't spell "world" backward or do a simple division, your blood sugar may be too low and you need to stop exercising immediately and consume some sugar (for example, an energy bar, or orange juice).

Be aware of your temperature and your sweating. Physical activity increases body heat production and core temperature, leading to greater skin blood flow and increased sweating. Your temperature regulation can be impaired if you have prediabetes or diabetes for many years. This can more easily lead to dehydration and even cause a drop in blood pressure if you get too hot or too cold.

I hope I'm inspiring you to incorporate exercise into your daily life. But don't overdo it. When exercise is done incorrectly or it's done too fast, injuries can occur. You want to progress slowly to minimize risk of injury.

A couple of other points to keep in mind:

- Always wear socks, preferably ones made with synthetic fibers, and athletic shoes that fit well and are comfortable. Don't try to squeeze in shoes that are too small. With exercise, form *over* fashion, please! ☺
- Always be on the lookout for blisters or cuts. Make it a habit to check your feet and hands after each workout. When these occur in persons with prediabetes or diabetes, they often get infected quickly. If you don't look, you may not notice until they are already too far along.

- Make sure you keep your skin dry. Exercise is going to cause sweat to develop. Too much sweat and heat on your skin for too long, especially around your feet and groin area, can cause fungus to develop. Don't be afraid to use powder in those areas.

Let's Get Started

Most people can safely start an exercise program. As noted earlier, I do recommend you discuss with your doctor before you start, especially if you have been sitting around a lot lately. Prolonged sitting can weaken your muscles, decreasing your fitness level, so you might need more help getting started. I am also a big supporter of using apps, online videos, virtual training, or even an in-person personal trainer for a period of time. It's important to exercise correctly and to have a program that fits your lifestyle. How many of you actually have an exercise *plan?* I bet many of you don't and that's part of the problem. As the saying goes, if you fail to plan, you plan to fail. I have gone to the gym and not been sure what I should work on many times. If I'm at home, I may have a break and decide, "I should exercise," and then I need to ask myself what exercise should I do. Without a plan, my workout is not well organized, doesn't work the body the way it should, and I don't get the benefit. Then I get frustrated that I'm not making progress!

I fixed that by doing some personal training sessions at a gym as well as using some online programs. Every Sunday I look at the week ahead to see when I may be able to do it. I'm flexible so if one day doesn't work, I fit it in on the next day. I don't "settle" for doing it just twice a week. And honestly, I notice a difference in how I feel on the days I engage in exercise. When you think about it, do you ever regret exercising? You probably feel pretty good afterward—and for several hours later.

To help you get started, I've included a four-days-a-week exercise program, covering four weeks. There's lot of different exercises to choose from. Of course, everyone is a little different but for those of you that need guidance early on, this provides a potential plan.

Summary

Start thinking about exercise as something you *need* to do instead of something you *should* do. To reduce your risk of prediabetes and diabetes, you should be trying to do 150 minutes of exercise every week, through a combination of cardio, resistance, and flexibility exercises. Some people might be able to save time by using high-intensity interval training to get the same benefit, if not more, in less time. Check out the various apps, online resources, and personal training services to help you develop a plan and perform the exercises correctly. And be sure to talk to your doctor about your plans.

ANSWERS

1. **TRUE.** Just fifteen minutes of daily exercise—if done in a way that requires exertion—can start you on the path to healthy living and reduce your risk of prediabetes and diabetic complications.

2. **FALSE.** Although cardio—or aerobic exercise—is important, lifting weights and flexibility exercises are equally important.

3. **TRUE.** Vigorous exercise lowers blood sugar.

4. **FALSE.** Building muscle does not replace fat. Muscle and fat are two different kinds of tissues and one doesn't replace the other.

5. **FALSE.** With some exceptions, most chores can be considered physical activity but would not be considered exercise without a significant amount of exertion.

CHAPTER SEVEN

The Distress of a Diagnosis

TRUE OR FALSE?

1. Diabetes increases your risk of depression.
2. Depression increases your risk of diabetes.
3. People with diabetes experience more problems with blood sugar control early on rather than years later.
4. Antidepressants are the best way to treat depression if you have diabetes.
5. Indulging in a few "cheat days" might help you control your blood sugar more easily.

(Answers at end of chapter)

YOUR BLOOD SUGAR AND your brain are connected in many ways. By now, you know the impact of prediabetes and diabetes on your physical health—but what about ways it affects your mental health? To maximize your physical health, you need to maximize your mental health. The mind and body are connected. Think about it this way—there is no physical health without mental health.

Being told you have diabetes—or even prediabetes—changes your life. This change can be hard. You need to adjust the way you eat, sleep, and exercise. Your daily routine is no longer routine—you have to completely revise it.

Some of you will need to check blood sugar daily. Most of you will have many more doctor appointments than you ever had before. Each visit reminds you of a chronic condition. It's physically and emotionally draining.

At some point, many of you will be feeling that you are losing control. There's a name for it: diabetes distress. It's what you feel when you simply are overwhelmed some days, when you feel like diabetes has overtaken your life. You have a job, relationships, responsibilities. Who needs more things to deal with? Sometimes people refer to it as burnout. It's quite common, and at some point, you will likely experience it. In any eighteen-month period, 33 to 50 percent of people with diabetes have diabetes distress.

These overwhelming feelings can be quite challenging and might lead you to slip into unhealthy habits. For example, you might skip doctor's appointments, stop exercising, discard healthy food options, stay up later than usual—all making your condition potentially worse and increasing your risk of complications. The consequences can be serious.

Diabetes distress impacts your body not just through the direct relationship with your self-care but by causing hormonal changes that can impact your diabetes. Stress, anxiety, and depression can cause insulin resistance. Recent research has shown how chronic psychological stress increases your body's levels of cortisol, the stress hormone, as well as inflammatory markers and chemicals called catecholamines. The presence of these chemicals circulating throughout your body keeps you in a state of constant stress—not something you want. High levels of cortisol cause the liver to create more glucose and keep your cells from absorbing glucose, allowing the glucose to build up in your blood. Essentially, this does the opposite of what insulin does. This buildup of high blood glucose, as well as the constantly elevated cortisol, means your body must secrete more and more insulin to clear the glucose out of the blood, resulting in insulin resistance over time. Worsening insulin resistance leads to worsening diabetes. Worsening diabetes leads to worsening diabetes distress, making everything worse. It's enough to make you throw up your hands and say "why bother?" Incredibly frustrating!

You might be surprised to learn that diabetes distress doesn't typically occur early on after diagnosis. Rather, we often see this in people whose feelings have changed over time, from first diagnosis to many months or a couple of years later.

I see something similar in patients who experience a heart attack. When first diagnosed, they are receptive to lots of changes. Everyone cleans out their pantry and starts exercising. But over the next few months, it becomes harder to maintain these changes, and people resume unhealthy habits. I often see patients who despite their initial desire to adopt healthy lifestyle changes, end up weighing more and having higher cholesterol levels years after their heart attack. It takes work to sustain change so that it becomes the new normal. And let's face it—that's not easy to do.

Signs of diabetes distress:

- Anger about your diagnosis
- Feeling alone
- Denying your condition
- Ignoring your feelings

- Frustrated about having to change your life to manage it
- Lack of motivation
- Feeling defeated and powerless
- Guilt if blood sugar numbers aren't good
- Fearful of diabetic complications and low blood sugar episodes
- Worrying about long-term effects
- Overwhelmed with what you need to do

You may have experienced some of these symptoms but didn't recognize them as signs of "distress" but rather just normal feelings of someone who has prediabetes or diabetes. "Doesn't everyone feel this way?" is often the response when I suggest people may need a little help. Let's be realistic. There are often ups and downs in your health journey, which can cause anxiety and stress. But it's important to acknowledge the severity and the impact of these feelings.

Depression Versus Diabetes Distress

If you have diabetes or prediabetes, it's understandable, and in some ways expected, if you experience some sadness or even depression. In fact, you are two to three times more likely to get depressed than people without diabetes. A recent study found that those who were newly diagnosed with diabetes were 30 percent more likely to have had a depressive episode in the prior three years. You may be wondering—if it's common to get depressed, does it really matter? The answer is *yes!* The impact of depression can be very real. Diabetes and depression together are more likely to cause disability or death than either disease on its own. Those who live with both are also more likely to have a lower quality of life and poorer glycemic control than those people with only diabetes. If you have diabetes and also experience depression, you are less likely to maintain an exercise regimen, stick to a prescribed diet, take medications, and check blood sugar consistently. In fact, one study showed that depressed patients missed double the number of doses of their diabetes medications than non-depressed patients.

Unfortunately, depression is often underdiagnosed and even misdiagnosed. This happens in people with and without diabetes. Only 25 to 50 percent of people with diabetes who have depression get diagnosed and treated. We need to change that. Diagnosis and treatment for depression is critical. Studies consistently show that people with depression and diabetes who were treated for their depression were twice as likely to get their diabetes under good control than those who did not get treatment. When it comes to using medication for depression management, it can be a little more challenging since some medications used to treat depression—but not all—can cause weight gain and therefore worsen insulin resistance, so discuss with your doctor which medications would be best for you. Untreated mental health issues make diabetes worse, and problems with diabetes can exacerbate mental health issues. If one gets better, however, the other often does too.

How to Know If You Are Suffering Distress

I do want to point out something very important—diabetes distress is not the same as depression. The feelings associated with diabetes distress may come and go, whereas with depression, the sadness and loss of interest are constant. In diabetes distress, you don't have those feelings about other parts of your life. You manage diabetes distress differently than depression, so making the distinction is key to effective treatment.

Diagnosis

One of the best ways to diagnose diabetes distress is through questions. There are several questionnaires that are helpful. Not surprisingly, some are called the Diabetes Distress Scale. There are different versions, typically with a range of three to twenty questions. Your health care provider should be screening for diabetes distress each year.

A common screening tool is called the PAID-5 (PAID stands for "Problem Areas in Diabetes"). This five-question assessment to gauge a patient's level of emotional distress includes statements such as "Feeling scared when you think about living with diabetes" and "Worrying about the future and the possibility of serious complications," and a range of possible responses with corresponding points: not a problem (0 points), minor problem (1 point), moderate problem (2 points), somewhat serious problem (3 points), serious problem (4 points). The higher a patient scores on this assessment, the higher their level of diabetes-related distress.

Unfortunately, not all doctors are good at screening for diabetes distress. I recommend you answer the questionnaire yourself and then discuss it with your health professional.

Too often, depression also goes undetected. Here's a good screening test that I often use. It's called the Patient Health Questionnaire (PHQ-2). It's two questions:

OVER THE LAST 2 WEEKS, how often have you been bothered
by the following problems?

1. Little interest or pleasure in doing things
    ❏ 0 Not at all
    ❏ +1 Several days
    ❏ +2 More than half the days
    ❏ +3 Nearly every day

2. Feeling down, depressed, or hopeless
    ❏ 0 Not at all
    ❏ +1 Several days
    ❏ +2 More than half the days
    ❏ +3 Nearly every day

Your PHQ-2 score is obtained by adding the number for each
question; your total will be a number from 0 to 6. Patients whose
total is 3 or greater, may be experiencing a major depressive dis-
order and should be further evaluated by a health professional.

Ways to Treat Diabetes Distress

Good news: numerous, effective treatment options are available
nowadays. Remember, it's important to distinguish if it's diabetes
distress or depression. One just can't treat any associated depression with drugs since it's multifactorial. Although some people
will benefit from antidepressants, those with diabetes distress can
benefit from learning coping and control skills.

What do I mean? We know that people with diabetes distress
feel that they have less control over managing their disease.
Patients who have a greater sense of control typically manage

their diabetes better; they adhere to lifestyle strategies and medication schedules better and, consequently, have a lower HbA1c. In other words, if you approach your diabetes management as being difficult and burdensome, it's more likely to be that way. If you approach it as being controllable and manageable, you're more likely to succeed.

Perhaps you are rolling your eyes, thinking, "Yeah, Dr. Whyte—I can just *will* my diabetes or prediabetes into control." Of course, it's not that simple, but I can offer some practical strategies that can help.

Strategies to tackle burnout and distress:

- Take time every week to do things you enjoy. It can be mentally and physically exhausting thinking about your health all the time. Make sure you find time to do things you like, whether or not they directly impact your health. Just do it because you enjoy it. Of course, that doesn't mean drink to excess or abuse substances. But maybe you like to play cards or listen to music. Gardening might be your source of joy. Maybe it's going out with a friend for coffee. The key is to spend some time every week that gives you joy.

- "Don't make the perfect the enemy of the good." I didn't always understand this phrase while growing up. Basically, this means you don't have to do everything right all the time. Some days your blood sugar will be good enough. And if you don't eat healthily every meal or miss an exercise session here and there, that's okay, as long as most days of the week you *are* doing the right thing. You don't have to follow guidelines perfectly to still reduce your risk of diabetes or prediabetes. All too often, the desire for perfection leads to an all-or-nothing philosophy: "I already ate donuts for breakfast, so, since I already blew my diet, I might as well eat candy the rest of the day." This ultimately creates more distress and worse blood sugar control.

- Give yourself a break. You might need to take a couple days to just reset. Of course, you don't want to let your blood sugar get out of control, but every now and then you might need to just take a day off and not worry about things. Just so you know—"every now and then" means every few months . . . not every week.

- Develop a support system of family, friends, colleagues, and health professionals that will be there when you need them. Look to family, friends, your doctor, and diabetes educators for support so that you don't have to figure it all out on your own. We have learned from the COVID pandemic that support systems can be virtual! Connect with other people with diabetes or prediabetes. Talk about how you feel and open up about your experiences and struggles with others who are going through the same. You'll find that you're not alone and may learn some helpful strategies.

- Embrace technology. If you are on medication and/or require use of a glucose meter, remote monitoring can make it much easier to obtain support from your health care team. One study evaluated a blood glucose meter linked to a smartphone-based app that automatically transfers a blood glucose log to your physician. In six months of using this device, the patients in this study reported significant satisfaction with their diabetes treatment, reduction in diabetes distress, and reduction in HbA1c. Physicians also had more reliable data more readily available to them and could intervene to change patients to a more effective diabetes medication if they noticed that the glucose values were too high. Another study looked at a virtual diabetes clinic that used smart devices to track blood glucose, as well as physician support and remote lifestyle coaching. After an average of six months participating in this virtual clinic, participants showed significant improvement in diabetes distress scores, especially those who had scored as "severely distressed" at the start of the study. Taking advantage of modern technology like this can help put you in greater control and simultaneously take some of the burden off you, therefore reducing your diabetes distress. Let technology bring care to you instead of you always having to go to the clinic.

- Pace yourself. Managing a healthy lifestyle often involves a lot of moving parts. Try doing one thing at a time, rather than tackling everything all at once. By breaking down your tasks into small bits and focusing on one or two goals that are easy to accomplish, you can minimize the discomfort of change, which can be distressing. Don't "bite off more than you can chew." If you haven't been exercising for a while, maybe start with one or two days a week instead of deciding that you are going to immediately start exercising five days a week. Gradually work up to your goal of three or four days a week. That way, you don't set yourself up for failure, and can celebrate success all along the way.

- Try yoga. If the thought of twisting your body into a pretzel makes you wince, consider the impact yoga has on your mind and body. It's all positive. It can help you re-center your thoughts and release endorphins, those feel-good hormones that reduce pain and promote happiness. At least one study has shown that people with diabetes who practiced yoga twice a week for twelve weeks lowered *both* their stress level and their blood sugar.

- Get a good laugh. They say laughter is the best medicine, so it's no surprise that studies have shown that laughing frequently can buffer your response to stress, probably by releasing serotonin, which can also help treat depression. In fact, laughter has also been associated with lower HbA1c. I agree the studies aren't the best designed, but it's worth a try, isn't it? The point is that laughing and joking creates happiness that can help address the distress of managing a health condition daily.

- Curb clutter. Messiness, whether in your home or office, is more than just an eyesore. It changes how we feel. Data shows visual chaos goes to your brain—overwhelming it with too many stimuli. When I look at my messy desk, it causes me anxiety—not knowing exactly where certain things are, and what I might need to be doing. (Don't ask me how it got that way!) Other times, I perceive clutter as a reminder of work that needs to be done—and hasn't yet been completed, resulting in some anxiety. Some neurologists believe the messiness distracts you and gets in the way of your ability to process information. (They studied it by looking at the MRIs of people's brains before and after clutter.

What would they see if they did an MRI of you?!) Although this doesn't directly impact your management of diabetes and prediabetes, it can still play a role in how willing you are to implement various components of a healthy lifestyle. Clutter contributes to distress.

Summary

Getting a diagnosis of prediabetes or diabetes stirs up a lot of emotions. How you feel about your condition makes a difference in how well you manage it. While some degree of frustration here and there isn't cause for concern, be alert for signs of burnout or diabetes distress. The more quickly you recognize the distress, the easier it will be to address it, and there will be less impact on your blood sugar control. Don't forget to make sure your doctor screens for diabetes distress.

ANSWERS
1. **TRUE.** People with diabetes are at increased risk for depression.
2. **TRUE.** Depression increases the risk of diabetes by more than 20 percent.
3. **FALSE.** Problems are more likely to develop in later years rather than at the time of diagnosis.
4. **FALSE.** Antidepressants may not be the best treatment option for depression associated with diabetes. Numerous non-pharmacological interventions have proven to be more effective.
5. **TRUE.** Taking a couple days off every few months might actually give you better control over prediabetes and diabetes.

CHAPTER EIGHT

Sleep Your Way to Better Blood Sugar Control

TRUE OR FALSE?

1. Lack of sleep can make you hungry.
2. Only too little sleep impacts your blood sugar.
3. You can catch up on sleep during the weekends.
4. Some people only need five or six hours of sleep.
5. Melatonin improves your sleep and your blood sugar.

(Answers at end of chapter)

PHYLLIS IS SEVENTY YEARS OLD and has had diabetes for nearly fifteen years. There are stretches of years where her blood sugar is under good control with lifestyle and medications, but during other stretches, it's not so good. Lately her HbA1c has been climbing up. "I'm really not doing anything differently, Dr. Whyte, so I'm not sure why that's the case." Her diet hasn't changed, and her activity level has actually increased. But her husband's sleep apnea has gotten worse. "I can't stand his snoring—I made him go into another room." And her knee pain has gotten worse. "Honestly, I'm not sleeping well. Is there anything you can give me?" was her recent request to me. Although we spent quite a bit of time talking about her blood sugar, she didn't make the connection to her lack of sleep and the change in her blood sugar control. She was treating her sleep issues as a separate problem and not one that could also be causing problems with her diabetes.

Patients are always surprised (sometimes irked or confused!) when I ask questions about sleeping. I tend to ask a lot of them, because I have learned how important your sleep quality is for your overall health. "I'm here to talk about my blood sugar!" is a common response. Most people aren't aware of the relationship between sleep and blood sugar. We all know that eating the wrong foods and being inactive can up your odds of developing diabetes. But did you know that lack of sleep is a risk factor for diabetes that is as important as being overweight, not exercising, or having a family history of the disease? Sleeping less than six hours a night increases your risk of diabetes by 20 percent. And if you're getting less than five hours of sleep each night, you're 40 percent more likely to develop the disease.

When it comes to diabetes and prediabetes, most people don't make the connection between sugar and sleep. That's a mistake.

Poor sleep isn't just a nuisance, it's an epidemic. The Centers for Disease Control and Prevention found that one in three adults fall short of the recommended daily amount of sleep. Quality sleep is a problem so prevalent that the federal government called it a national health priority that needs to be addressed as part of its Healthy People 2030 initiative, in part because of the impact that it has on diabetes rates.

When it comes to diabetes, one obvious problem with a lack of sleep is that you don't feel like eating well or exercising when you're exhausted. And when you're tired, you're certainly more prone to high levels of stress. We know that these components can impact blood sugar, so it's easy to see how a chronic lack of sleep can add up to trouble when it comes to diabetes.

But sleep's effect on diabetes goes much deeper than that.

The number of hours you sleep and the *quality* of your sleep impacts your diabetes risk. Researchers studied more than four thousand people who reported how much sleep they got each night. Those who got less than six hours were twice as likely to have cells that were less sensitive to insulin or to have full-blown diabetes. This was true even after the researchers took other lifestyle habits into account.

But how does insufficient sleep directly influence the development of diabetes? On its face, the relationship might not seem intuitive, but your sleep habits can either protect you from diabetes or predispose you to it. We have a growing body of research showing the relationship between lack of sleep and diabetes risk, including large studies that have tracked thousands of people for decades—looking at how much they routinely slept and how that impacted their health outcomes. After decades of research, we now have a clear understanding of how sleep loss affects your hormones and blood sugar levels, your immune system, your appetite, and even your brain function. You might be surprised by what you're about to read.

Sleep and Insulin Resistance

HOW LACK OF SLEEP AFFECTS BLOOD SUGAR

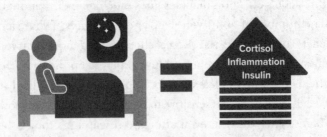

As you now know, in type 2 diabetes, your body doesn't respond as well to insulin. We have also learned in recent years that insulin seems to operate on a daily cycle. By that I mean there are times throughout the day when our cells are more and less sensitive to it. When you disrupt your circadian clock by cutting back on sleep or adopting an irregular sleep schedule, it throws your system out of whack. The cells in your pancreas experience stress, leading to dysfunction, and other tissues throughout your body become less sensitive to insulin. This has a direct effect on your blood sugar levels. In a recent study, scientists found that when they restricted a group of healthy young adults to just four hours of sleep every night for one week, they experienced a sharp decrease in their glucose tolerance, which can signal the onset of prediabetes. The subjects also had higher overall blood sugar and insulin levels, and tests showed that they had become less sensitive to insulin. But amazingly, their glucose tolerance returned to normal when they were allowed to sleep for nine hours a night over the next six nights—showing that sleep could be both the cause and the cure to their blood sugar problems. Multiple studies have replicated these findings, which is pretty strong evidence that when you skimp on sleep, you may be putting your body on a path toward becoming insulin resistant. And it doesn't necessarily take years either. Although it is not a true comparison, animal studies have found that just one night of sleep deprivation can impair insulin sensitivity as much as six months on a junk food diet!

Sleep and Inflammation

When you lose sleep, you throw your immune system into overdrive, causing it to churn out higher and higher levels of powerful immune cells that promote inflammation. It's as if you're sending your body's army out to battle, but the problem is that it ends up launching friendly fire on your own cells and organs. We've known that chronic inflammation is a major contributor to your cancer risk, but we now know it also affects your diabetes risk. When you lose sleep, an inflammatory molecule known as interleukin-6, or IL-6, becomes active. In clinical studies, scientists found that when they forced healthy adults to sleep for just four hours a night—down from their usual eight hours— for twelve nights in a row, their bodies produced up to 62 percent more IL-6 compared to when they slept normally. In the real world, scientists found something similar in night shift workers: their bodies secreted higher levels of IL-6 at night, when they were up working instead of sleeping.

But IL-6 isn't the only molecule that causes problems. Sleep loss causes your body to ramp up its release of many other inflammatory agents, including tumor necrosis factor α, also known as TNF-α, and c-reactive protein, or CRP. One study found that for every hour of sleep that you lose, your body produces about 8 percent more TNF-α. Sleep deprivation has a similar effect on CRP, a protein made by the liver that can signal that your body is fighting off an infection or dealing with widespread inflammation in your veins and arteries. Taken together, what we know is that the less time you spend in bed, the more you push your body into a heightened state of inflammation, creating a "storm" of immune cells that can wreak havoc on your body, particularly when it comes to diabetes risk. One study showed that people who had higher levels of IL-6, CRP, and other inflammatory markers were two to four times more likely to develop diabetes compared to people with normal levels of these compounds. And that was after the researchers accounted for factors like age, BMI, and whether the participants smoked.

Insulin plays a big role when it comes to inflammation. It turns out that insulin has other jobs besides stimulating your cells to take up glucose. It also has the ability to fight inflammation. As sleep loss creates higher levels of inflammation, your body releases more insulin, and eventually becomes less and less sensitive to it. That helps to drive a vicious cycle that accelerates your path toward insulin resistance.

Cortisol

When we talk about sleep and diabetes, it's important to talk about the role of cortisol. Normally, our bodies follow what is called a diurnal pattern of cortisol production. That means cortisol levels rise in the morning as you wake up, which gets you alert and ready for the day, and then taper off in the latter half of the day as you wind down and get ready for sleep. When you lose sleep, your body produces higher levels of cortisol. Studies have found that a night of too little sleep causes cortisol levels to remain elevated throughout the day, especially in the evening. This causes problems: it increases glucose production, lowers glucose uptake in your peripheral tissues, and reduces insulin secretion. Cortisol also pushes your body to store more fat. So, over time, with consistently poor sleep, heightened levels of cortisol will chronically raise your blood sugar levels and increase your body fat. One recent study recruited thousands of healthy adults in England and tracked their cortisol levels over several years. It found that people whose cortisol levels tended to remain elevated in the evening—instead of tapering off—were significantly more likely to develop diabetes or prediabetes in the decade that followed.

Melatonin is a hormone in your blood that plays a critical role in maintaining regular sleep patterns and in keeping your circadian clocks synchronized, but it also appears to affect insulin. We've known for several years that certain gene variants associated with melatonin receptors are strongly linked to higher risks for type 2 diabetes. Recent research has shown that if your melatonin level is high, it may reduce the ability of insulin-making cells in the pancreas to release insulin—and that people with those genetic variants experience this insulin-suppressing effect more strongly.

Leptin and Ghrelin

Two other hormones that play a role in whether you may develop prediabetes or diabetes are leptin and ghrelin. These hormones play two very different roles, and they tend to move in opposite directions. The first one, ghrelin, is nicknamed the hunger hormone because it motivates us to eat. Ghrelin is produced in the stomach and small intestine. When it's released, it travels through the bloodstream to a part of the brain that governs appetite, where it triggers hunger. Think of ghrelin as a hungry little gremlin that periodically emerges from hiding in your stomach to demand that you feed it. Ghrelin makes you consume more calories and then store that food as fat. It served a role to prevent starvation thousands of years ago, but nowadays when it is out of whack, it can make us fat.

It's not just the weight gain from ghrelin that increases diabetes risk. When ghrelin rises, it causes our glucose levels to increase too. Scientists have found that when they administer ghrelin to healthy young adults it causes an immediate spike in their blood sugar levels and worsens their glucose tolerance, which can increase the risk of prediabetes. This may have been another evolutionary adaptation that served our ancestors well. When food was scarce, ghrelin would spike, pushing them to hunt and forage while simultaneously keeping their blood sugar levels from plummeting to dangerously low levels.

But now that we only have to take five steps to our kitchens to fix ourselves a meal, rather than running for five miles to catch a gazelle, we don't need ghrelin flooding our bodies. That is one reason good sleep is so important. Numerous studies have shown that getting enough shut-eye helps to keep ghrelin in check. Other studies have found that sleep restriction prompts spikes in ghrelin, especially in the morning. That's why sometimes you wake up famished!

The other part of this story is leptin—the yin to ghrelin's yang. Leptin is the so-called satiety—or satisfied—hormone. It tells our brains when we are full, letting us know it's time to put down the fork and step away from the table. But when leptin levels fall, we can have a hard time knowing when to stop eating. In fact, people who have leptin deficiencies suffer from chronic overeating and uncontrolled weight gain. Leptin also plays a role in our glucose metabolism. Scientists have found that administering leptin directly lowers blood sugar and insulin levels. It has also been shown to improve insulin sensitivity, helping your body to function more as it should. Sleep deprivation suppresses leptin production. In fact, multiple studies have found that when people are limited to just four hours of sleep a night, their leptin levels plummet nearly 20 percent. Large observational studies of thousands of people have also found that short sleepers have chronically low leptin levels.

Please recognize that sleep can have a big impact on your risk of developing diabetes (and your ability to control it if you're already diagnosed). Although you may have previously thought that missing some sleep isn't a big deal, I hope you are now seeing that it is critically important when you want to reduce your personal diabetes risk.

I know people want to "average" their sleep over the week—catching up on the weekends. I'm sorry to tell you it doesn't work that way. The studies consistently show that it's the quality of your *daily* sleep that determines your diabetes risk. And if you are already prediabetic, lack of sleep may be contributing to your condition. All of this drives home a crucial point. What you do at night has just as much impact on your diabetes risk as what you do during the daytime—so sleep wisely!

And for those of you who think more is better, this might disappoint you: recent research suggests that getting too much sleep also has negative effects on insulin sensitivity and glucose tolerance. The key is getting the right amount of quality sleep.

How Do You Know If
You're Not Getting Enough Sleep?

The simplest way to determine how well you're doing with your sleep is to simply ask yourself: "Do I feel rested and refreshed when I wake up in the morning?" If the answer is no, you likely need more sleep. Do you set an alarm? If you do, how often do you hit the snooze button? If it's most days of the week, you need more sleep.

For those of you that like data, you also can use trackers on your smartwatches, phones, and even your bed and pajamas to tell you if you're getting a good night's sleep! I went to the Consumer Electronic Show a few years ago and it was all about high-tech mattresses and pajamas that monitor your sleep. (Yes, many people do wear pajamas!) I do think those are helpful to look at, especially the trends over time. I have been using one over the past year and there is a good correlation between how I feel in the morning and my sleep score. Even more so, when I get a "low score" indicating poor quality sleep, I renew my efforts to get better sleep. That's what I find is the best aspect of these trackers—continuous feedback.

If you're willing to do a sleep experiment, I have a good idea to help you learn how much sleep you need, no matter your age. It's called a "sleep vacation." The name is a bit misleading since, as I mentioned, it's more of an experiment than a vacation. This is an especially good test for those of you who rely on alarms.

Here's how it works. You need to pick a time over a two-week period when you don't need to wake up at a specific time, since for this "vacation" you are not going to use an alarm. You won't count the first two or three days because you will likely be anxious there's no alarm. Go to bed the same time every night and allow yourself to wake up naturally. Over those two weeks, you will develop a pattern of sleeping that's likely around eight hours, plus or minus an hour. There are some people—very few—who have a "short sleep phenotype" that allows them to function efficiently with only five hours of sleep, with no harmful effects. Don't assume, though, that you have that phenotype!

Getting Quality Sleep Is Key. So How Do You Get It?

If you're like most people, you are sleep deprived—as those gadgets, tools, and experiments may have confirmed. Now what do you do?

I don't want you to rush to sleep medications, which is what many people do. Those medications have a role, but I do think they have been overprescribed. They were designed for short-term use—and while everyone expects to take them for only a couple of days, folks often end up using them long term, for months or even years. There's a real concern they disrupt normal sleep patterns. The same for supplements—people start to use these as a "crutch" that they need for good sleep. Sometimes it starts as just needing some sleep before an important work assignment, and then it quickly becomes something they need every night. Once that happens, it gets very difficult to stop them.

The most effective solution to sleep problems is something you may have never heard of (and doctors rarely discuss)—cognitive behavioral therapy (CBT). This approach involves identifying and then addressing factors that cause insomnia, including the sleep environment. It helps to address and change your sleep behaviors. It takes time and work, but there's good data supporting its effectiveness.

Most experts suggest CBT should be used *first*—before you even try medications. Unfortunately, most of us don't really try it. It's a multicomponent therapy, typically done over four to eight sessions with the help of a physician or therapist. It consists of the following components:

- Sleep restriction
- Sleep compression
- Stimulus control
- Sleep hygiene
- Counter-arousal measures

Sleep Restriction Therapy

The name is a little misleading because it doesn't aim to restrict actual sleep time but rather to initially restrict the time you spend in bed. You basically try to limit the time in bed to only sleep time. At first, it deprives you of sleep so that you create a situation where your body thinks "sleep" when your head hits the pillow. You start off by reducing the amount of time in bed so by the time you go to bed you will be sleepy. Subsequent steps consist of gradually increasing the time spent in bed.

For example, consider a person who goes to bed at 11:00 p.m. and gets out of bed at 8:00 a.m. but sleeps on average only six hours per night. During the first step of this procedure, this person will be in bed only six hours (for example, between 12:00 a.m. and 6:00 a.m.). This sounds harsh but after a week or so there will be a marked decrease in time spent awake in the middle of the night.

The next step is to gradually extend the time spent in bed by fifteen- and thirty-minute increments, as long as the number of episodes waking up in the middle of the night remains minimal.

This can be tough to do and should be done under a doctor's or therapist's guidance, but many people do eventually achieve restful sleep.

Sleep Compression

Sleep compression is an alternative to sleep restriction. It is a slightly different technique with a gentler approach. It's often a better option, especially for older people. Instead of immediately reducing time in bed to the amount of sleep you get on a typical night, you gradually decrease it until it approaches the time you spend actually sleeping.

Sleep compression includes gradually compressing bedtime over several weeks to approach the sleep time you registered during the first week of treatment.

Stimulus Control

Stimulus control therapy is based on the theory that you have become conditioned to sleeplessness. Now you need to relearn an association between your sleep environment and rapid sleep onset. Stimulus control involves a set of instructions that are designed to eliminate situations in which you struggle in bed and increase the frequency of falling asleep quickly.

- Establish a regular time you get up in the morning. Routines help strengthen your circadian clock, which regulates sleep and wakefulness. This can be hard early on since it can be difficult for some people to fall asleep around the same time every night. That's why you need to keep at it, partly to reset your circadian rhythm.

- Go to bed only when sleepy. Seems pretty simple, but it can be hard to differentiate between fatigue and sleepiness. Fatigue is a state of physical or mental low energy. Often, someone will say, "I feel tired." Sleepiness is a state of having to struggle to stay awake. Dozing off while watching TV or as a passenger in a car involve sleepiness. You might say, "I can't keep my eyes open." People with insomnia often feel tired but "wired" (not sleepy) at bedtime.

- If you're unable to fall asleep, either at the beginning or in the middle of the night, get out of bed and return to bed only when sleepy again. You might have to do this a couple of times early on.

- Try to eliminate any napping. If you need a snooze, make it quick—typically around ten or fifteen minutes and definitely not more than thirty. Don't do it past 2:00 p.m. or 3:00 p.m. Anything later than that is going to disrupt your normal sleep, messing up the routine we are trying to establish.

Sleep Hygiene

It's not an elegant term, but basically "sleep hygiene" interventions involve targeting behavioral habits that negatively impact sleep. Some of these are incorporated into the other components as well:

- **Make your sleep space into a spa.** Your bedroom needs to be dark, quiet, and cool. Have you ever gone to a spa that is bright and loud? I bet not because they wouldn't be in business for very long. I will admit that spas are usually warm, but when it comes to your "sleep spa," lower the thermostat. The data show that most people sleep better in cool temperatures. The ideal temperature? Sixty-seven degrees. I know that the thermostat is often a battleground in the bedroom, but cooler is better. Give it a try and see how your sleep goes.

- **Wear socks to bed.** Not exactly what you suspected, is it? Wearing socks in bed increases blood flow to your feet and causes heat loss through your skin. That lowers your core body temperature. The role of socks and sleep is a little bit counterintuitive, but there is science to support it.

- **Hang some room-darkening shades.** I must tell you they can work wonders. There are different levels of darkening, and you may lose some of the light cues for awakening if no sunlight at all can get through in the morning, but many people find success with these shades. For the same effect, you can just wear a sleep mask over your eyes. It keeps out the light, and many people say it helps signal their brain, "the day is over—it's time for sleep." It can take a couple of nights to get used to masks, so be sure to try it more than just once or twice.

- **Decrease sound.** Consider that your brain still hears and processes sound while you sleep. That's the reason why you want the room to be quiet. The sounds that your brain hears can wake you up, even from deep sleep. Some of my patients use earplugs and others use white noise machines. Personally, I just try to keep the room quiet.

- **Use a humidifier.** Whenever I mention a humidifier to patients, they usually seem to think it's something that's in a museum! "Do they still sell them?" is often the reply! Using a humidifier puts moisture back in the air and can make it easier to fall and stay asleep. Humidifiers are particularly useful during the winter when the air is often dry. Dry air can cause irritation in mucosal membranes in the eyes, nose, and throat. They also help in the summer when allergies can cause a cough, which can keep you up, or when too much air-conditioning also makes the air dry. Use distilled water if you can get it—it works best. Just be sure to clean your humidifier every day.

- **Consider your bedding.** When did you buy it? Have kids been bouncing on it? Does it sag in some places? Most experts recommend you change at least every ten years, preferably sooner. Mattresses lose their shape and firmness over time. Have you ever "sunk into" a mattress? It's not comfortable. I'm sure some of you are using the first mattress you ever bought. They can get expensive, I know, but sleeping on an old, worn-out mattress is not only bad for your back, it's bad for your sleep. My mother often complained of back pain, and, in retrospect, I think her mattress contributed to it.

  What kind of mattress is best? For the best sleep, your mattresses should evenly distribute pressure across your body. Firmness is a matter of personal preference. Be sure to turn the mattress 180 degrees every six months or so. That way, you don't only use one section of the mattress. Be sure to get some help, though, when turning it. It's harder to do than it seems! A good friend of mine shared some advice over two decades ago that's good to repeat: "John, you spend a third of your life in bed. It's the one place you spend the most time in your life. Get a comfortable mattress."

Examine those sheets too! I'm not talking about thread count, although 300 to 400 would be a good goal. The key is to not forget about changing and cleaning them. Body oils, dead skin cells, and perspiration linger in your sheets. Bacteria and dust mites also accumulate. Some people suggest your sheets have more germs than a toilet seat! All of this can cause irritation to your skin and throat, worsening conditions such as asthma and eczema. It's hard to sleep when you are itchy. Most experts suggest cleaning at least every two weeks.

Ever try a weighted blanket? There are a wide range of quilts and comforters on the market now that can weigh between five and thirty pounds. This extra weight seems to provide a gentle pressure that can give the feeling of being held. Some data suggests this type of pressure can cause the release of serotonin, a neurotransmitter that helps promote sleep. I have tried these blankets and do think they can help with sleep.

For me, the most important part of the bed for good sleep is my pillow. The pillow for your head should support the natural curve of your neck and be comfortable. Many of us have our head and neck too high or too low on the pillow. A pillow that's too high can put your neck into a position that causes muscle strain on your back, neck, and shoulders; one that's too low causes hyperextension. The pillow should maintain a height of four to six inches to support the head and neck (and shoulders when lying on the back).

Some people suggest sleeping with no pillow. I am not a fan of this approach since it can eventually cause neck pain if there is poor alignment. Basically, it comes down to personal preference. If you have trouble sleeping or wake up with neck, arm, or back pain, experiment with a different pillow as well as how high you lie on it.

My wife sprays lavender on her pillow. Some data suggest aromatherapy increases deep sleep, perhaps by slowing heart rate and lowering blood pressure and temperature—which can help one feel more rested. It might be worth a try! You can even try an air diffuser in the bedroom.

- **What about pets in your bed?** Good news! Allowing your pet to sleep in your bed can help with sleep. Studies show that having a dog in the bed can help relieve insomnia by lowering anxiety and modifying your threshold for waking up. A dog's rhythmic breathing, when one lies next to you, can help lull you to sleep. Cats help too. Many cat lovers talk about how the purring sound soothes them. Pets in the bed might even increase flow of oxytocin, another "feel-good" hormone. Just remember to clean the sheets a bit more often.

Hide Your Phone, Pad, Tablet, Computer

How many of you use the time when you get into bed to catch up on your social media, or just to "go over emails." Bedtime is not the time or place for social media catchup or other screen time. Remember, you want to quiet your mind when you prepare to sleep. How often does email or a social media post create an emotional response from you? That's not what you want before sleep. Almost everything we do on phones and tablets is stimulating to our brains, especially social media, texting, email, and online shopping.

How many of you put the phone on your nightstand? Do you set it to sleep or airplane mode? If not, make sure your phone goes to sleep when you do! No email or text will be so urgent that you need to keep your phone right by you. If that's really the case, you can allow certain numbers to still ring through the sleep mode. Don't be a "JIC-er"—those folks who want to keep it nearby "just in case." I always ask people "just in case" what? They don't usually have a practical answer! A friend of mine puts her phone in the closet before she goes to bed. I know most of you aren't probably willing to do that—she says it takes a few days to get used to, but she swears she sleeps better and is less stressed every morning. It might be worth a try!

Is Your Light Blue?

The other problem with screens before bed is blue light. I have had patients say their screens don't emit blue light, but it's not a light color we can see with our eyes. Blue light is a wavelength emitted from many of our digital devices. It turns out some of the energy-efficient lighting we all have become enamored of also increases our exposure to blue light. The problem with blue light is that it can suppress the body's release of melatonin, making it more challenging to fall asleep because your body thinks it's time to wake up. Some good news—nowadays, new devices have been designed to emit less blue light. But, even if you use a newer device, it's still a bad idea to use it before bed.

What about those fancy blue light–blocking glasses? The American Academy of Ophthalmology does not recommend spending money on blue light glasses to improve sleep. Rather, they suggest simply decreasing evening screen time and setting devices to night mode.

Bottom line: I recommend you turn off all screens an hour before bedtime.

Check Your Meds

Medications are one of the top disruptors of sleep. I'm not talking here about sleep medications (which will cause sleep disruption in the long run) but rather those other medications you may take—both prescription and over the counter—that may impact your ability to get a good night's sleep. For instance, within the last few years, there has been a trend—supported by data—to take medicine for high blood pressure in the evening, rather than in the morning. Since some high blood pressure medicines have a component of a diuretic—you end up having to get up at night to urinate. Other medications known to impact sleep include:

- Steroids, including prednisone
- Inhalers
- Diet pills
- ADHD drugs
- Anticonvulsants
- Some antidepressants

Nonprescription drugs that can cause sleep problems include:

- Pseudoephedrine
- Drugs that contain caffeine, including some cough and cold medications
- Illegal drugs such as cocaine, amphetamines, and methamphetamines
- Nicotine, which can disrupt sleep and reduce total sleep time; smokers report more daytime sleepiness than do nonsmokers, especially in younger age groups.

Don't stop any of these prescribed medications without talking to your doctor. Sometimes sleeping issues caused by these medicines may be solved by changing the dose or the time of day you take them.

Caffeine

What's the skinny on coffee? The data describing caffeine's impact on sleep hasn't been consistent. In theory, caffeinated beverages block a brain chemical called adenosine, which promotes sleep. In practice, while some studies do show that coffee makes it harder to fall asleep, others say it has no effect. I enjoy coffee, especially in the morning. I rarely drink it in the evening, but I have on occasion without consequences. That's just me; many friends and family members can't have a cappuccino after dinner unless it's decaf (by the way, decaf coffee still has some caffeine!). I recommend you test yourself. If you have a cup after 3:00 or 4:00 p.m., and it keeps you up, then make it a point not to have caffeine past noon.

Try to Relax

The last component of CBT is counter-arousal measures—this typically means relaxation techniques. Two common approaches are progressive muscle relaxation (PMR) and diaphragmatic breathing.

- **Progressive muscle relaxation.** PMR involves tensing and relaxing different muscle groups in the body over about ten seconds, focusing on getting into a relaxed state.

- **Diaphragmatic breathing.** Diaphragmatic breathing is a technique focused on longer breaths that balance oxygen and carbon dioxide levels to bring your body to a state of relaxation. Since anxiety is associated with faster, shallow breathing, this type of breathing from the diaphragm or belly rather than the upper chest can help bring a sense of calm.

- **Mindfulness.** Several of these practices can help you get ready for sleep and even maintain sleep. They help address the anxiety that may be preventing you from getting restful sleep as well as "quieting your mind," stopping it from racing with different thoughts. The coronavirus pandemic accelerated the development of several good apps to help guide mindfulness sessions. There are a lot of free ones as well as trials. Examples include Calm, Headspace, Buddhify, and Smiling Mind. I do recommend to most people that they try an app or some type of guided session the first few times. There's a process to effective mindfulness and it's good to practice it.

Avoid Looking at the Time

One thing we all experience is waking up and then getting anxious about the time. When we look at the clock and worry about how much sleep we are losing, that only adds to our stress. And makes it harder to relax and get back to sleep. We've all been there—"It's 3:00 a.m. and I'm not asleep yet!" One solution is to turn your clock toward the wall or put your phone in a drawer.

Staying Up Late as Revenge Bedtime

I recently learned about the concept of revenge bedtime procrastination. This is the idea that with all the stress and overworking we do, putting off bedtime is a way to reclaim some time for yourself. You're going to stay up late to "still enjoy the day" after working so hard. The problem is you often cut down on your sleep by doing this. A better strategy might be to try to carve out thirty minutes during the day where you feel that time is yours. Maybe it's going for a walk, talking to friends, or reading a book.

Summary

Your sleep and your blood sugar are connected. If you want to reduce your risk for prediabetes and more effectively manage diabetes, please don't ignore the quality of your sleep. You can't eat healthily, exercise five days a week, and then only sleep six hours a night. It will negate many of the good things you are doing. If you are trying hard to manage your diabetes or prediabetes and you are having trouble, poor sleep may be the cause. Getting quality nightly sleep needs to be a priority and not something you relegate to the weekends. Be sure to review your medications and the time you are taking them with your doctor. Ask your doctor if some of the components of CBT may be something you should try.

ANSWERS

1. **TRUE.** If you don't get enough quality sleep, it will cause disruption of key hormones that can make you hungry.
2. **FALSE.** Both too little and too much sleep can cause problems with blood sugar control.
3. **FALSE.** There's no catchup of sleep on weekends. It's what you do on a nightly basis that matters.
4. **TRUE.** There are some people—very few—who can function well on five or six hours a night.
5. **TRUE.** Melatonin in our body can help with sleep and blood sugar control.

CHAPTER NINE

Stress Busters That Help You Manage It All

TRUE OR FALSE?

1. Any amount of stress raises your blood sugar.
2. Chronic stress triples your risk of prediabetes.
3. Listening to music can reduce your stress.
4. Stress is always bad for you.
5. If you are stressed, you will feel it.

(Answers at end of chapter)

"I WORK FULL-TIME, and I've got two young kids at home, and, honestly, don't have a lot of support. I'm doing the best I can, Dr. Whyte." This was Sarah's immediate response when I mentioned her blood sugar had been higher than usual. I barely got beyond that statement when Sarah also remarked, "And my parents are having their own health issues, and they live halfway across the country. I've got a lot going on." Sarah is right—she has a lot going on. More and more people are juggling multiple priorities. For many people like Sarah, this causes stress. Like most people with diabetes or prediabetes, Sarah doesn't realize that her stress is also making her blood sugar harder to control— for a variety of reasons that I will explain.

Stress is a major factor in diabetes. Stress prompts our bodies to release chemicals that raise your blood sugar; and when we feel stressed, it makes it harder to maintain healthy eating habits, sleep eight hours a night, and exercise thirty minutes most days. And if that's not enough, working to manage your diabetes can create even more stress! It becomes a vicious cycle. Learning how to manage stress in your life plays a major role in you being able to take control of your prediabetes and diabetes risk.

Let's talk about how our bodies respond to stress and how it affects our health.

You've probably heard the expression "too much of a good thing"—stress is one of those things. Yes, stress *can* be a good thing. Stress can prompt us to action. Many of us find that we think more clearly, and work more efficiently, when we're under a little bit of pressure. That's because our bodies are hardwired with a stress management system.

When your brain encounters stress, it triggers a response that evolved over millions of years to ensure human survival. This response was critical for our ancestors. It ensured that when they encountered a predator or a rival from a neighboring village, they had the ability to stay and fight or turn and flee—the so-called "fight-or-flight" response. Our stress response was a way to stay alive! But the world is very different today—with other types of dangers! And the dangers we face today don't resolve as quickly as the physical dangers our ancestors faced— stressors like an overly demanding job, a bunch of bills piling up, or a toxic relationship may last for years! And this is a problem because our stress response system was designed as a burst of energy to get us out of immediate danger—it wasn't designed to stay on *all the time.* When our stress response is constantly activated, it can do damage to our bodies. Our stress response is a double-edged sword—one that has the power to both protect us *and* put us at risk of developing prediabetes as well as cardiovascular disease and other chronic health conditions when it goes haywire.

Here's how the stress response works. When you encounter a threat (a tiger . . . or a toxic boss), a tiny, almond-shaped structure in your brain called the amygdala registers it. The amygdala processes emotions like fear, and when it detects a threat it instantly alerts another region of the brain called the hypothalamus, which tells the body what to do. Think of the amygdala as the lookout in a patrol tower that sees an army of invaders approaching. It alerts its general, the hypothalamus, which rouses the troops and prepares them for battle. The hypothalamus activates the sympathetic nervous system and sends a signal to your adrenal glands, which quickly unleash hormones such as adrenaline into your bloodstream. This accelerates your heart rate, dilates your pupils, raises your blood pressure, increases your pulse rate, and prepares your lungs to take in more oxygen—all the things that your body needs to fight off a tiger or run at top speed. I bet you have all felt this at work in your life—when you were scared late at night or before an important presentation. This is very helpful in brief situations, but when stress becomes chronic and these hormones remain elevated, problems arise.

Why is this the case?

Our brains interpret a lot of stressful stimuli as a threat, like an overbearing colleague, rush-hour traffic, or the loss of a job. Even an unhappy relationship or the grief and despair caused by the death of a loved one can trigger this response. When these things cause you to experience persistently high levels of stress and anxiety, your brain gets stuck on high alert. This puts your body in a chronic state of fight-or-flight mode—which is not what nature intended. After a while, it takes a toll on your health—including how your body manages your blood sugar.

Stress and Diabetes: The Physiological Mechanisms

When your brain is constantly on high alert due to chronic stress or anxiety, it activates what is known as the hypothalamic-pituitary-adrenal axis, or HPA, a feedback loop between organs involved in the fight-or-flight response. One role the HPA plays is to instigate the release of the stress hormone cortisol, which directly influences your diabetes risk. Cortisol belongs to a class of hormones known as glucocorticoids, which get their name from their ability to increase glucose levels. As we discussed in previous chapters, cortisol mobilizes your body's energy stores, causing a flood of glucose and fat to pour into your bloodstream so you have an immediate supply of energy—glucose—to take action against whatever threat you may be facing.

When you're under a lot of stress, your cortisol levels spike, driving your liver to ramp up its production of glucose. Over time, if cortisol is constantly elevated, your blood sugar will be constantly elevated as well. Persistently high levels of cortisol and other glucocorticoids can also cause your cells to resist insulin, accelerate the breakdown of muscle tissue, and increase visceral fat, which is the kind that accumulates around your internal organs, deep in your belly. One recent study found that people who have persistently elevated cortisol levels are more likely to develop prediabetes and diabetes throughout their lifetimes. Other studies have shown that cortisol is tightly linked to blood sugar levels. In healthy adults, cortisol levels are supposed to fluctuate throughout the day—rising in the morning and then falling in the evening in alignment with our circadian rhythms. But people with diabetes whose cortisol levels remain elevated throughout the day have higher glucose levels—and the smaller the drop in their cortisol levels from morning to night, the higher their average blood sugar levels. One study found that people with diabetes who have consistently high levels of cortisol secretion had more frequent and severe complications from the disease, such as kidney problems and nerve damage.

SHOULD I ASK MY DOCTOR TO MEASURE MY CORTISOL LEVEL?

Cortisol levels vary throughout the day. They go up and down based on a variety of factors. The tests we have right now aren't sensitive enough to provide useful information about stress. Cortisol levels may give us useful information about other conditions but they can't determine whether you are too stressed.

Like stress, the problems with cortisol start when there's too much of it. Cortisol is helpful to our bodies because it has powerful anti-inflammatory properties. Ordinarily it reduces inflammation and suppresses the immune system. This is a good thing when cortisol spikes in response to an acute but temporary form of stress that requires your body to focus its resources on survival. But again, when cortisol remains elevated for prolonged periods, the immune system starts to become *resistant* to it, leading to a sort of rebound effect that results in inflammation throughout your body. Studies show that people with chronically elevated cortisol tend to have high levels of inflammatory markers, such as CRP, IL-6, and TNF-α—all of which are associated with an increased risk of developing diabetes. Some experts have even characterized diabetes as a chronic low-grade inflammatory state—which acknowledges the relationship of your stress levels and your ability to control your blood sugar.

Another consequence of chronic stress is that it impacts your blood pressure and heart rate, which can then affect your blood sugar. You might be thinking—*we are talking about prediabetes and diabetes, not hypertension.* True, but there's a connection. Remember how I mentioned that the "fight-or-flight" response constricts your blood vessels and spikes your heart rate? This raises your blood pressure, pushing blood and nutrients toward the core of your body. That's great if you're faced with a life-or-death situation. But when chronic stress raises your blood pressure time and time again, it can increase your risk of diabetes. Researchers recently tracked 4.1 million people over a period of roughly seven years. At the start of the study, none of the participants had diabetes. But the researchers found that people with high blood pressure were most likely to go on to develop the disease. In fact, an increase of 20 mm Hg in systolic blood pressure was linked to a 58 percent higher risk of developing diabetes. Another study of 120,000 people found that the higher your resting heart rate, the greater your risk of developing diabetes. Every ten-beat-per-minute increase in resting heart rate was associated with a 19 percent higher risk of the disease. Of course, there are other factors in play, but it's clear that elevated blood pressure and heart rates can impact your diabetes risk. If you suffer from both, your risk of complications from either increases dramatically.

We've Known but Ignored
for Centuries the Effect of Stress

You're probably saying, "I never knew this about stress and blood sugar." The reality is that we've known for centuries that they are intertwined—we've just done nothing about it. As far back as the seventeenth century, British physicians noted that the development of diabetes seemed to be driven by what they called "prolonged sorrow." We noticed a similar situation a century or so later with a condition in medicine known as "broken-heart syndrome," in which grief, sadness, and other types of emotional pain cause a person's heart to weaken and change shape. Time and again, when scientists have studied large populations, they have found strong evidence that high levels of stress seem to drive the development of disease.

Stress Changes Your Behavior—
And Not in a Good Way

Stress not only drives up your blood sugar directly, it also contributes to the other factors that increase diabetes risk. People who struggle with high levels of stress can be less motivated to exercise or eat a nutritious diet. I bet when you are stressed you aren't too worried about whether you are eating healthily or finding time to go to the gym. Being stressed changes your behavior. For instance, people with chronic stress often smoke and drink more and engage in other unhealthy behaviors as coping mechanisms. But even after researchers control for these factors, the link between stress and diabetes remains very strong. Recently, researchers followed thousands of industrial workers, looking at how their experiences at work impacted their long-term risk of developing disease. They found that people who endured high levels of work stress—especially those who felt that they put in a lot of effort for very little reward—had as much as a 26 percent higher rate of developing prediabetes and up to a 27 percent higher risk of diabetes in the years that followed. A separate study followed more than 2,500 people over five years and found that a higher incidence of stressful life events and chronic psychological stress was strongly linked to diabetes. People who had the highest rate of stressful life events were a staggering 60 percent more likely to develop diabetes, even after the researchers controlled for things like socioeconomic factors, a family history of diabetes, poor diet, and sedentary behavior.

If you're a woman, you may be at particular risk. Scientists recruited about 3,800 women and analyzed their overall health, including giving them tests to evaluate their glucose metabolism. Then they followed the women for five years and documented their exposure to stressful events like the death of a loved one, financial hardship, or the breakup of a marriage. At the end of the study, the researchers found that women who experienced more of these events and who reported higher levels of perceived stress were most likely to develop prediabetes. This occurred in a "dose-response" relationship, meaning the higher the level of stress, the greater the risk of developing the disease.

I could fill the next ten pages with more studies, but I think you see my point. Chronic stress is an important factor for you and your doctor to consider when you are looking at your personal risk for prediabetes and diabetes. Recognizing when you are experiencing chronic stress and controlling or even eliminating the sources of it in your life may be one of the best things you can do to protect yourself from diabetes.

Lessening the Effects of Stress in Your Life

Managing your stress will help you control your risk for prediabetes, and if you have diabetes, could prevent complications. We know that eating healthily, exercising, and getting restorative quality sleep are all important to addressing stress and keeping blood sugar and insulin under control.

What else can you do? I often suggest a two-pronged approach. One is to try to minimize the effects of stress in your life, and the second is to learn to manage your response to stress. Because stress is such a big factor—affecting directly and indirectly your ability to implement the other changes I suggest in this book—it's critical that you have useful tools. But you first need to recognize that you are stressed and it's impacting your health. Remember, we all have some stress; it's the daily chronic stress that some people experience that causes the problems.

How Do You Recognize If You Are Stressed?

Everyone reacts a little differently. Some people experience an increased heart rate, while others experience headaches and trouble concentrating. Still others suffer problems with queasiness in their stomach and might start having diarrhea. Still others feel pain, particularly in the shoulders and neck. It's important to try to recognize any physical cues. It's also helpful to learn how you perceive your life. The way our bodies and our minds respond to an event or problem often depends on how we perceive it. Recognizing our perception of stress in an important first step.

I'm a big supporter of questionnaires when it comes to determining your stress. It's important, though, to use those surveys that have been validated—meaning they have under-gone study to prove their reliability. Some of these are admin-istered directly in a health professional's office and others are ones that you can do yourself. They are great self-assessment tools. The way you take control starts with recognizing what you need to take control of!

You should consider taking the Perceived Stress Question-naire. It consists of thirty questions and takes about fifteen to twenty minutes to complete. The scoring looks at your feelings of stress over the last year as well as over the last thirty days. It asks you to rate the frequency of feeling rested, irritable, lonely, overtasked, frustrated, tense, judged, mentally exhausted, as well as safe and lighthearted.

There's also the Perceived Stress Scale. It asks about feelings and thoughts during the last month. It's only ten questions and focuses on how often you get upset or feel you are unable to control important things or feel angry or believe that things aren't going your way.

Some people might be so stressed, they can't even focus on the questions. If that's the case, consider this single question: Is your stress giving you an edge or getting in your way?

Depending on the results of your stress inventory, some of you will need professional help to help you manage your chronic stress. Most people will be able to make some simple changes and find relief. The following are some suggestions to help you manage stress and ultimately help with your blood sugar control.

Try to Stay Positive

It may seem cliché. And you might be thinking, *Really? I just need to think positive thoughts and my life will get better?* No one thinks it's that simple, but science does show the role that our

STRESS BUSTERS

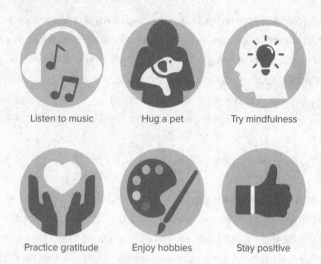

Listen to music   Hug a pet   Try mindfulness

Practice gratitude   Enjoy hobbies   Stay positive

attitude has on our physical health. Some studies have shown that the impact of how you perceive stress—is it enhancing or debilitating to your health—affects how your body and mind respond. Researchers looked at the mindset, stress perception, and success of Navy Seal candidates. Those that viewed stress as positive did better in the training, had faster times in physical challenges, and received higher reviews. I'm not suggesting that you view all sources of stress as positive because many are definitely not. But your perception and attitude play a big role. And you want to be careful not to have a "woe is me" approach either. Let's be realistic—it may require some practice. In the exercise chapter, I talk about how muscles grow when they are stressed. Positive thinking becomes a habit and grows through practice—often during difficult times.

Try to Practice Gratitude

Find something to appreciate in each important area of your life, such as your family, friends, work, and health. That perspective can help you get through tough times. Every week, try writing down three things you are grateful for but also why you are grateful for them. Forcing yourself to write it down will make you think about it and that can help address stress.

Accept What You Can't Change

Growing up, I learned a prayer attributed to St. Francis of Assisi that many people know as the "Serenity Prayer." It speaks to changing the things one can, accepting those that one cannot, *and* the wisdom to know the difference between the two. The last part is what's so hard for many of us. We may not be able to change our circumstances, but we can change our perspective and our reaction.

Set Boundaries

It's okay to say no to things that you don't really want or need to do. If you find yourself saying yes to a lot of things you'd rather not be doing, it might be time to start boundary setting. Boundary setting plays an important role in helping you and others understand what you can and cannot do. In many ways, it's about transparency—to yourself and others. Be sure to ask yourself whether it's worth saying yes. If you can develop a framework to help you assess activities, that can help reduce your stress. Realistically, you will be putting more emphasis on your needs and feelings than those of others—but hey, that can be a good thing to do!

Be Kind to Yourself

Do you expect too much from yourself? We need to learn to be kind to ourselves. We treat others with compassion, and we also need to show self-compassion. Release yourself from self-criticism. Too often, we traumatize ourselves with our own unrealistic demands to succeed—*we* become our sources of stress. Be on the lookout for those overly critical thoughts and slowly replace them with thoughts of encouragement. "I know I'm doing the best I can."

Stop Multitasking

I know people like to brag about how many things they can do at one time. I suggest you stop the juggling. Several studies have shown that if people attempt more than two tasks at once, their focus suffers and stress levels may increase.

Try Mindfulness

I mentioned this earlier. People often feel more relaxed after some deep breathing and guided imagery. Research supports that people with diabetes who practice mindfulness can lower their blood sugar. Remember, try some apps or directed instruction. Mindfulness takes practice to get the benefits.

Listen to Music

Relaxing music can ease anxiety. I know some doctors use music therapy to help treat anxiety and stress in cancer patients. What's been particularly compelling is a study that showed merely listening to music has a calming effect—and those persons who said that their specific purpose in listening was to relax showed a significant decrease in anxiety and stress levels measured by self-assessment, cortisol, and other biomarkers! I suggest that you make a playlist of your favorite stress-busting songs but keep it as a separate list from some of your other music. And don't worry if you don't like classical music—even those quick-tempo pop and dance songs can help calm you after a few minutes of listening. Heart rate and blood pressure do go up initially but go down when the music stops.

Hug a Pet

Interacting with pets has been shown to reduce cortisol levels. Some experts suggest that because pets are nonjudgmental, they may help buffer your response to stress. We certainly saw how pets helped people with anxiety and PTSD during the recent COVID pandemic. Numerous studies have shown that being a pet parent lowers blood pressure, and dog ownership seems to increase life expectancy. (We are still waiting on cat data. ☺) If you're not ready for a pet full-time, you can volunteer at a shelter or even be a foster-pet parent.

Hobbies

Fight stress by forgetting about it. Lose yourself in a favorite pastime. Do something that relaxes you, like reading, playing a musical instrument, gardening, or painting. When was the last time you played a board game with family or friends? I would caution you, however, not to make a hobby a new source of stress. I have friends who used to love golf, and then they began to get very competitive. Eventually, they were no longer having fun golfing, and managing all the different practices and tournaments just became too much.

Volunteer

You might be thinking, *I'm stressed enough. I don't have time to help others. I have to help myself.* Well, maybe you can do both through volunteering. There's a fair amount of research that shows when we spend some time helping others, we focus less on our own stress and problems. Maybe it's something you could start trying once a month.

Let That Grudge Go

We've all had a situation that did not go our way or a had a family member, friend, or coworker mistreat us. Scientists have found that holding a grudge and the associated anger can continue to increase our stress. There's a tool that some therapists use named with the acronym REACH: Recall the hurt, Empathize with the one who mistreated you, Acknowledge that this was something that hurt you and you have the right to be hurt, Commit to then letting it go—knowing that it is a gift you are giving yourself— Hold on to that gift, and do not allow that painful emotion to live in your mind. Buddha said, "Holding on to anger is like drinking poison and expecting the other person to die."

Summary

Stress is a natural part of life, and our bodies are created to handle it—in *temporary* doses. But when stress becomes constant, the mechanisms designed to keep us healthy start having an oppo-site effect. Ongoing stress causes multiple health problems, in-cluding difficulty in getting your blood sugar under control. To stay healthy—and to take control of your diabetes risk—it's vital that you develop a keen awareness of the amount of stress in your life. Talk to your doctor and use questionnaires to get a realistic view of your stress level, and then TAKE ACTION by implementing strategies to get stress under control. You can start slow, adding one stress relief practice at a time (managing stress shouldn't become a *source* of stress). I understand you may feel like you have too much on your plate already and can't possibly add stress management to your to-do list—like the pa-tient I mentioned at the beginning of this chapter—but the health risks are simply too serious to ignore. So spend some time noticing the stress in your life, and then decide what you can do to take control.

ANSWERS

1. **TRUE.** Any amount of stress can raise your blood sugar.

2. **FALSE.** Chronic stress doubles your risk of prediabetes.

3. **TRUE.** Listening to music that you enjoy can reduce your stress.

4. **FALSE.** Some stress is necessary for survival. It is the daily, chronic stress that starts to cause disease and decrease the quality of your life.

5. **FALSE.** When stressed, your body gives off clues. We often don't recognize the symptoms of stress and attribute them to other sources. Part of the goal of this chapter is to help you recognize the physical and mental impacts of stress.

CONCLUSION

It's a Journey

IF YOU'VE EVER BEEN ON a road trip, you know that you must make a lot of preparations before you hit the road, and that your work continues during your journey. It's the same when you are told you have prediabetes or diabetes—you need to figure out what steps to take to get you to where you want to go and what resources you'll need along the way—and then you need to make sure to stay on course. It's what comes next that matters the most. You can't change the past, but you can influence the future by taking control of your risk.

As you set out on your health journey, here are a few things I think you should consider.

Who's your copilot?

Just as you carefully consider who will be part of your road trip crew, you should choose your diabetes crew carefully.

And when it comes to who should ride "shotgun," your doctor plays a key role.

I encourage people to periodically evaluate their relationship with their doctor. I know many patients who stay with a doctor that they don't have the best relationship with just because it's the easiest thing to do. "It's too difficult to find a new doctor" or "they're all the same" are typical responses when I ask people why they didn't switch when they expressed unhap-piness with their current physician. The reality is that your doc-tor is your copilot—doctors play a key role in your health so you need to have a strong relationship with them.

How do you tell if it's the right fit? Here are a few factors to keep in mind:

- How easy is it to get an appointment and communicate with your doctor? Given the role of telemedicine as well as numerous messaging apps, you should not have to wait weeks for an appointment or days to get your questions answered. If they're that busy, you need to assess whether you are getting the attention you deserve.

- Are your labs explained and do you have access to the full report? I'm not a fan of doctors simply saying "your labs are normal" or "everything is fine" or "it's a bit high." Your doctor should go over the numbers and what they mean—whether they are normal or abnormal. You should also have full access to your lab reports.

- Do you feel your doctor listens to your concerns and considers ideas you have? I encourage patients to tell me what they are reading online or what they are hearing from friends. If you have questions about supplements, your doctor should take the time to answer them. If you want to know if it's worthwhile to try intermittent fasting or whether you should try an app that measures body fat, you should be able to discuss it without fear that your doctor will be dismissive. I've tried to answer a lot of the questions I get from patients in this book, but your doctor also needs to engage with you on your concerns about your health and your ideas. You are trying to take control of your risk and your doctor needs to be an active participant.

- Sometimes you need to be referred to a specialist, and your doctor should be willing to make that referral. Some doctors, either because of professional pride or payment incentives, don't refer patients to specialists as often as they need to. If you want a second opinion or feel you need to see a specialist, your doctor should help facilitate it.

If you aren't getting what you need, then yes—you should get a new copilot.

Your "diabetes crew" may also include family members, work colleagues, or friends, and you may share your diagnosis with them, but that's totally up to you. You may not want to share your diagnosis with everyone in your life, and that's okay. Who to tell is a decision that may take some time to make, and everyone is a little different. Basically, you need to ask yourself if sharing your prediabetes or diabetes diagnosis with someone is going to help you in your efforts to reduce your risk or possibly make it harder. I've mentioned throughout the book the importance of support. I'd suggest you tell people who you believe will offer that support and help you reach your goals. We don't need people to blame us or make us feel guilty. You also don't want someone who, despite their best intentions, becomes the "diabetes police" and nags you about every daily decision you make. Most of the time, family members, spouses, roommates, and friends can help on your journey. They might even make it more interesting! It can be an opportunity for everyone to get healthier.

Check the Tires

When you go on a road trip, you check the tires and make sure you have enough gas. Do the same thing when you begin your journey to reduce your risk of prediabetes and diabetes.

If you've been told you have prediabetes or diabetes, you need to be getting a yearly physical. Some of you will need visits more often, especially if your blood sugar is not well controlled. Remember, having elevated blood sugar puts you at risk for many other health conditions, including high blood pressure, high cholesterol, and heart disease. Getting data—lab tests, vital signs, physician exam—will help you stay on course as you go about your diabetes journey. I mentioned that many times people don't go back to their doctor after they are told they have prediabetes or even diabetes. Please don't be that person. If you don't take active steps to adopt healthy behaviors, your diabetes can worsen and complications can develop.

You also need to get your eyes checked. Remember, one of the first complications of high blood sugar is damage to your vision. Getting your eyes checked out on a regular basis is key to keeping them in good working order. When we were growing up, my sister always used to say "I swear on my eyes" when she wanted me to believe something. Our vision plays a critical role in our quality of life. Please don't compromise it.

Pay attention to your feet. Chronically elevated blood sugar damages the nerves and decreases the blood circulation. Keep your toenails trimmed and consider moisturizing a few days a week. Be on the lookout for bruises or changes in color or temperature. Although you might love flip-flops, it's not a good idea to drive in them and not ideal to wear them all the time even during the summer. Wearing them all the time can damage your bones and tendons as well as cause more blisters and injuries.

Focus on your mouth. Not just what you eat, but also your teeth and gums. I know I'm asking you to see your doctor *and* your dentist, but as I mentioned earlier in the book, diabetes increases your risk of dental problems. Just as you wouldn't want problems with your car's air-conditioning while you were on the road, you don't want problems with your mouth as you try to make healthy lifestyle choices.

Get up to date on vaccinations. Having diabetes can decrease your immunity, so it's even more important that you make sure you are fully protected. Many vaccines are determined based on age, but the presence of diabetes may make you eligible for vaccines earlier than expected. Both the CDC and ADA recommend the flu, hepatitis B, Zoster, Tdap, and pneumonia vaccine.

Finally, do not smoke. I've had patients over the years tell me that smoking helps them keep off the pounds. While weight management is an important component in reducing diabetes risk, the damage done by smoking far outweighs any perceived weight benefit.

How Will You Handle Detours?

Trips don't always go exactly as planned, do they? Occasionally you have to take a detour, either because of traffic or you saw some cool little shop you want to check out. Well, managing prediabetes or type 2 diabetes is a trip where there will be bumps and detours on the way. You may get injured during your exercise program; you may experience a life event that creates more stress; or you may experience a health complication. When those detours occur, it can be very discouraging and frustrating, and it can be difficult to get back on track.

Encountering detours on road trips can create opportunities: you may find a quicker route than GPS suggests, or you may run across a shop with just the earrings you've been looking for. The same goes for the detours along your diabetes and prediabetes journey. You may realize that intermittent fasting works better than trying to eat oatmeal every morning. You may try yoga to recover from an injury and discover you love it! My point is that there's no one way to get healthy and you should try different strategies. Patients will often tell me they "tried something and it didn't work." I always try to refocus the discussion on what we can find that *does* work. Journeys are about looking *forward*—and that's what you need to do when there are setbacks. Of course, we learn from the past and try not to make the same mistake twice, but if one method isn't working to lose weight, you need to try another.

At some point, you may be put on medication. That doesn't mean you should stop incorporating lifestyle changes. I've seen quite a few people over the years think that starting insulin means they can become lax about their healthy eating habits. I expressed a bit of surprise with my patient Barbara, who told me she has a cupcake treat several times a week. "It's okay, Dr. Whyte. I just take a little more insulin and my sugar is fine."

Other patients have a different view—they see starting medication as some sort of failure. But please know that taking metformin or other medication is not a bad thing—it can be a very important step in your health journey. You also don't want to compare your journey to others. Everyone is on a different path, and what works for someone based on genetics and their underlying health may not work for someone else.

We started off by talking about how being told you have pre-diabetes or diabetes is a wake-up call—signaling a need to take action. Over the past nine chapters, you've empowered yourself with the knowledge to take control of your risk.

Here's what I hope you have learned:

- There's no special prediabetes or diabetes diet. Rather, it's about treating food as medicine. Eat plenty of fish, fruits and vegetables, low-fat dairy, and whole grains while cutting back on processed meats, sugar-sweetened beverages, and refined grains.
- Create a love affair with exercise—more than just physical activity—that will not only help treat your diabetes but a range of other health conditions as well. If you can't exercise thirty minutes most days of the week, you might be able to do high-intensity interval training, which can give as much benefit in half the time.
- Recognize the importance of quality sleep. Sleep—preferably seven or eight hours a night—needs to become a priority if you want to control your blood sugar.
- Managing diabetes can cause distress and it is important to recognize the signs and symptoms. Make sure you get screened for diabetes distress.
- Our mental and physical health are connected, and you can't have one without the other. We all have stress in our lives. Some stress is good but daily, chronic stress makes it hard to take control of your blood sugar. Practical tools exist to help you limit stress to a healthy amount.

Yes, change is hard. It takes time, as well as a commitment. But the benefits are well worth it. Create the healthy habits you've been reading about. They will not only help you return your blood sugar to normal but also increase the quality of your life!

You have the power to take control of your risk. Start using it!

ACKNOWLEDGMENTS

EVER SINCE I WAS IN medical school, I've enjoyed learning about the diagnosis and management of diabetes. I'm grateful to all the professors I've had the opportunity to learn from over the years. I'm also enormously appreciative of all the patients I have worked with over the past two and a half decades. You've taught me as much about managing diabetes as I have taught you.

This book would not have happened without Mel Berger, literary agent extraordinaire at WME. Mel took the idea I had about a book on prevention and crafted it into a three-book series. He's kept me quite busy, but I am enormously appreciative of his counsel.

My friends at Harper Horizon—Andrea Fleck-Nisbet, Amanda Bauch, and John Andrade—have been trusted partners throughout the process. They're always supportive, always encouraging. I know they want the best content because we share the belief that better information leads to better health.

It seems like I've had an army of folks to help me out. My WebMD colleagues—Dr. Michael Smith, Dr. Brunilda Nazario, and Dr. Neha Pathak—ensured that I covered the most up-to-date research. WebMD and Medscape's Director of

Communications, Patricia Garrison, always gets the word out about what I'm writing, so we can maximize the reach.

Dr. Christopher Mohr helped shape the meal plan, and we had some provocative discussions about certain foods! I've known Chris for nearly fifteen years and appreciate both his nutrition knowledge and culinary prowess. Greg Herrell helped me think through an exercise program—my personal one—as well as the general principles that people with prediabetes and diabetes need to follow to maximize their health.

I appreciate the hard work of the illustrator, Sandra Bruner, who helped bring my words to life. A picture truly is worth a thousand words. Huge applause for my friend and colleague Kim Richardson. She has been involved with this book every step of the way. She challenges me to become a better author, and ultimately a better communicator. She has the nicest way of helping me write and rewrite content by making sure I use plain language and not lapse into medical jargon. I could not have gotten this book done without her help.

My sisters, Charlene and Jackie, gave me great advice throughout as I thought through different chapters. If you want unvarnished advice, ask a family member! Their comments helped to make this a better book.

Special thanks to my wife, Alisa, who is always a good sounding board for ideas.

My two sons, Luke and Jack, are still too young to read this book. Yet they provided the fun breaks needed to help restore my creative juices for some marathon writing sessions. I can't wait until they "stumble" upon this in a bookstore. Of course, I may guide them in the right direction!

Exercise Plan

EXERCISE NEEDS TO BE PART of your personal prevention program for both prediabetes and diabetes. It will be very hard to take control of your risk without exercise. One of the biggest challenges is getting started and knowing what to do. Everyone's interests and abilities are a little different, but the following four-week program helps you get started. There are a variety of exercises to consider as you develop a program that works for you.

The structure of the plan is as follows: four days total, including two days of cardiovascular and flexibility training and two days of resistance, core, and balance/stability training. Be sure to incorporate rest on those days when you aren't exercising. Your body needs time to recover and reset to get maximum benefit.

Week 1, Day 1:
Resistance Training/Core/Balance

Squat. These can be done with just bodyweight or if you're feeling strong you can hold a dumbbell at your chest (one hand on either side)—or even some books or a milk jug if you're around the house. When you're starting out, use a chair or couch as a target—to squat down to a consistent depth.

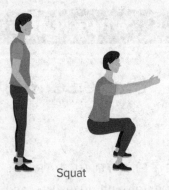

Squat

Pro Tip: To make the challenge even more difficult, slow your tempo on the way down, resisting for three to four seconds as you descend.

Sets/Reps: 3 sets of 10 reps

1. Stand with feet at or around shoulder width, toes straight and forward.
2. Drive your hips back, bending at your knees and keeping your knees from collapsing.
3. Sit into a squat position, imagining you're sitting down into an imaginary chair while still keeping your heels and toes on the ground, making sure to try to keep a neutral spine position.
4. Try to descend to the point at which knees are bent to a ninety-degree angle if there is proper form and no pain at that point.
5. Press into your feet and push using your quads to return to a standing position.

Alternative Lower Body Exercise

Reverse Lunges. If squatting is painful, or you just simply want some variety, you can replace squats with reverse lunges. Reverse lunges work similar muscle groups but also add a new element of stability.

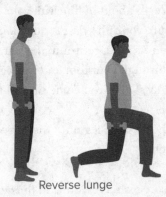

Reverse lunge

Pro Tip: Take off your shoes and socks for natural stability and to prevent the soles of your shoes from interfering with your mind-muscle connection. Add weight to your hands if you feel you need further resistance.

Sets/Reps: 3 sets of 8 to 10 reps on each side (do one side at a time)

1. Stand tall with your feet about shoulder width apart.
2. Keeping one leg planted, take a big step backward with your other foot while simultaneously lowering your hips and knee toward the floor.
3. Make sure you keep your spine in a neutral position by holding a straight upright posture in your back. Lower yourself toward the floor so that your back

knee lightly taps the floor or gets within about one inch.

4. You know you're in a good position when your knee is almost down or all the way down and the bent leg is close to or at ninety degrees. To help check if you're in a good position, make sure that the knee in the bent leg is about in line with your toes.

5. Making sure your hips don't rotate and your lower back doesn't round, return to the starting position by pushing through your foot and raising your hips and torso fluidly so that you come up and forward at the same time.

6. Repeat on the same leg until the reps are completed, then switch.

Bird-Dog. This core exercise is done in the quadruped position, meaning you'll be on your hands and knees. I'd recommend doing this on a rug or carpet. The key here is to create tension in your core the entire time you're performing the exercise.

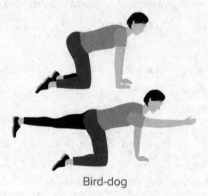

Bird-dog

Pro Tip: Try placing a tennis or lacrosse ball on your lower back and try to keep it from falling the entire time you're performing the movement to know you're keeping a neutral spine position.

Sets/Reps: 3 sets of 8 reps on each side

Rest after the second exercise as needed. Shoot for thirty to ninety seconds.

1. Begin on all fours with your hands directly under your shoulders and your knees directly under your hips.
2. Create tension in your core, pretend to grab the floor, and corkscrew your hands clockwise. Without moving your torso, push back into your toes to create further core tension. Keeping your back and pelvis still and stable, reach your right arm forward and left leg back. Stay as stable as you can, hold for one second.
3. Return to the starting position by placing your hand and knee on the floor. Repeat the same thing on the other side.

Push-Up/Incline Push-Up. Depending on your strength and mobility levels, you can make these as difficult or as easy as needed.

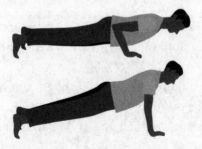

Push-up/Incline push-up

To make it more challenging, change the tempo during the up or down portion of the exercise. To make it more manageable, change the angle of the push-up: the higher, and more acute the angle in general, the easier it will be to perform. Use a wall, a table, a countertop, or some type of sturdy furniture.

Pro Tip: To help reduce the possibility of pain, keep your arms in a neutral position, meaning your elbows stay tucked in close to your body and don't flare out during the exercise. Also, as you lower yourself, make sure your elbows are not less than a ninety-degree angle relative to your body.

Sets/Reps: 3 sets of 10 reps

1. Get on the floor on all fours, positioning your hands underneath or slightly wider than your shoulders.
2. Extend your legs back so that you are balanced on your hands and toes. Feet should be shoulder width apart. Body is in a straight line from head to toe without sagging in the middle or arching your back.
3. Contract (create tension), corkscrew your hands into the ground clockwise, push back into your toes, and brace your core (imagine what you would do with your body if you were outside in a hurricane; get tight!).
4. Inhale as you slowly bend your elbows and lower yourself until your elbows are at a ninety-degree angle.
5. Exhale and push back up through your hands to the start position. Control your body through the movement; don't let gravity do part of the work for you.

Alternative Upper Body Exercise

Triceps Dips. Another way to target your pecs and triceps is using the triceps dips exercise.

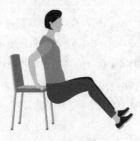

Tricep dip

Pro Tip: If your own body weight isn't enough, you can add weight like books to your lap to increase resistance.

Sets/Reps: 3 sets of 10 to 12 reps

1. Find a sturdy table or a step to serve as a base—it should be about hip height tall.
2. Place your hands, palms down and fingers pointing toward your body, on the edge of the base.
3. Walk your feet out until your legs are straight and balance on your heels so that your toes are lifted off of the ground.
4. Keeping your elbows tucked in close to your body, lower your entire body until your elbows are behind you at about ninety degrees.
5. Once at the bottom, briefly pause for no more than half a second and then return to the starting position by again keeping your elbows tucked in and

       straightening those elbows until they are almost
       completely but not quite locked.

6.   Squeeze your triceps at the top for no more than half
       a second and then immediately repeat.

Single Leg Barefoot /Stability Balance. The single leg barefoot
balance can be varied depending on skill level. Balance on one
leg barefoot as opposed to in shoes for greater mind-muscle
connection. Try closing your eyes and/or moving the opposite
leg clockwise around your body while remaining balanced on
one leg.

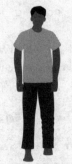

Single-leg balance

Pro Tip: You can also increase difficulty by changing the material (safely) that you balance on, whether that's a foam pad
or a pillow or whatever else you can find that you feel comfortable using.

**Sets/Reps: 3 sets of thirty seconds of balance
on each leg**

Rest after the second exercise as needed. Shoot for thirty to
ninety seconds.

1. Find a safe area, perhaps a rug or carpet, with plenty of room.
2. Balancing on one leg, lift the opposing leg just an inch or two off the ground.
3. Think about grabbing the floor with your foot to create greater stability through the rest of the body.
4. Start with thirty seconds on each leg and increase baseline difficulty as needed, whether that's adding extra time, closing your eyes, changing the surface you're balancing on (using a foam pad), and so on.

Horizontal Row. For those of us who sit all day (often hunched over), or even those who don't, it's important that we incorporate our "pulling" or back muscles into our routine. Examples of items to use are a gallon jug of water, or a light (five- to ten-pound) dumbbell.

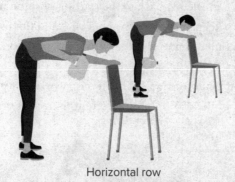

Horizontal row

Pro Tip: Remember, you can always change the tempo of the exercise, slow it down, increase the time under tension, and make the exercise more challenging.

Sets/Reps: 3 sets of 10 reps on each arm

1. Using a chair or table, find a surface that is stable and about as tall as the height of your navel or hips.
2. Place one hand flat on the surface.
3. Hinging at your hips and keeping a neutral spine (straight back), bend over until your flat back is about forty-five degrees relative to your hips.
4. With your opposite hand, grab the "weight" of your choosing; in this example, it's a gallon jug of water.
5. Keeping your back at the forty-five-degree and neutral position, "row" the jug of water to your torso making sure your elbow gets to a position of ninety degrees and making sure to keep the elbow close to the body.
6. Pause for half a second and then extend your elbow and lower the jug back to the starting position making sure to keep your torso from moving and not using any momentum to jerk the weight into position.

Body Weight Glute Bridge. This exercise works our glutes and hamstrings while also helping to strengthen and protect our

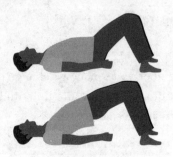

Glute bridge

lower back. The glute bridge requires no equipment, just a comfortable area to lie on your back.

Pro Tip: Do this exercise on one leg to increase the challenge and bring a little more core into play!

Sets/Reps: *3 sets of 10 reps on each leg*

Rest after the second exercise as needed. Shoot for thirty to ninety seconds.

1. Lie flat on your back with your knees bent.
2. Bring your heels toward your butt until they're about eight to twelve inches from the edge of your butt.
3. Making sure your feet are flat on the ground, push through the soles of your feet and extend your hips upward until they are about forty-five degrees relative to the ground.
4. Squeeze your butt cheeks together hard at the top and pause for one second.
5. Lower yourself back down slowly, count to two before your butt hits the ground again.
6. Repeat.

Week 1, Day 2:
Cardiovascular Training/Flexibility

Aerobic exercise. Thirty minutes of aerobic exercise. The importance of working your heart and lungs cannot be overstated. Whether it's walking, jogging, swimming, boxing, or cycling, the important factor is making sure the difficulty is moderate to vigorous, which will be different for every person and relative to your current fitness level.

Choose a moderate-intensity exercise today like a brisk walk, and make sure to go for at least twenty to thirty minutes straight.

Pro Tip: Monitor your heart rate as you go, if possible, to find out what heart rate zone you were in!

Wall Hamstring Stretch. Lots of people have tight hamstrings and hips, especially after working out. It's good for those with diabetes or prediabetes to couple their balance/stability training with some flexibility training as well.

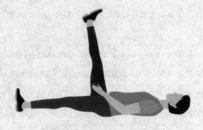

Wall hamstring stretch

Sets/Reps: 2 sets of 45 seconds on each leg

Rest after the second exercise as needed. Shoot for thirty to ninety seconds.

1. Find the corner of a wall that's sturdy enough for your leg to push against.
2. Lie on your back facing the corner of the wall; one leg is straight up against the wall, right at the corner, so that the other leg can rest flat on the floor.

3. Push your body toward the wall until you feel a moderate stretch in the back of your quad, aka your hamstring.

4. Pull your toes toward your shin to accentuate the stretch.

Cat-Cow. Helps to mobilize the thoracic spine, improve posture, and increase upper body mobility.

Pro Tip: You can also do this on a table or bench, if being on your knees is painful.

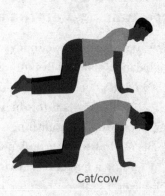

Cat/cow

Sets/Reps: 2 sets of 10 reps
(1 rep is going through 1 cat and then cow position)

1. Start on your hands and knees with your back flat and spine in a neutral position.

2. Hands are directly underneath your shoulders and knees are underneath your hips.

3. Push into your hands, rounding your back as far as you can while keeping your hands on the ground. Final position looks like you have a hunch back (or

scared cat). Hold for one second then move toward the next position.

4. Retract your shoulder blades, inhale, and pull your spine downward as you allow your spine to move in the opposite direction. In the final position your back looks like a "U." Hold for one second then move toward the next position.

Week 1, Day 3:
Resistance Training/Core/Balance

Split Squat. A nice way to work your lower body while also combining an element of balance/stability. By putting the emphasis on one leg at a time, you don't need as much added load to get the same training effect that a bilateral (or dual-limbed) exercise would. Meaning, depending on your fitness level, starting with assisted split squats might be plenty difficult. Assisted split squats can be done by finding a fixed object to use for support while you perform the exercise. If you're more highly trained, try slowing down the tempo and/or holding dumbbells or similar weighted water jugs in each hand.

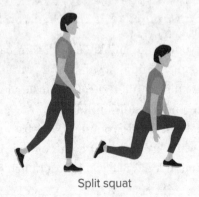

Split squat

Pro Tip: Elevate your back leg to put even more weight onto the working leg.

Sets/Reps: 3 sets of 8 reps on each leg

1. Placing one foot forward and one foot backward, the heel of your back foot should be raised so that you are balancing on your toes.
2. Making sure you keep an upright torso and being careful not to hyperextend, slowly lower yourself to the ground.
3. Finish right before your knee touches the ground or lightly tap your knee before returning to the starting position. Make sure you choose an appropriate resistance; form matters here, and if you can't maintain a rigid torso throughout the movement, it may be time to dial back the difficulty.

Seated Neutral Shoulder Press. Grab some light dumbbells, or water jugs, canned goods, water bottles, or paint cans. Just do your best to make sure they are identical or at least very similar in weight.

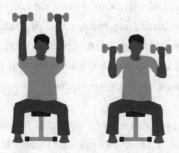

Seated neutral shoulder press

Pro Tip: We are going to start with the neutral position because it's often more comfortable for the shoulder joint.

Sets/Reps: 3 sets of 10 reps

1. Sit on a bench or chair with your feet flat and comfortably on the ground; make sure you have good posture.
2. Sitting up straight and keeping a neutral spine, raise your dumbbells or whatever household items you chose so that they are now shoulder height.
3. Keeping your elbows tucked in so that they run parallel to the sides of your body, press the objects overhead, fully extending your elbow.
4. At the top, a good check to make sure you're in a good position is to see if your biceps are in line with your ears.
5. Slowly lower the objects until your elbows reach about ninety degrees and then press back up again using control and making sure to stray from using momentum to help.

Hinge. A lot of people think about deadlifting, but no one should deadlift until they master the proper mechanics of a hinge and have the range of motion required to pull a barbell from the floor. A hinge can be done with your body weight, but making sure we're using proper form and sequencing here will be the key.

Pro Tip: Once you feel you've mastered the body weight hinge, try implementing a Romanian Deadlift. Find a balanced object like a kettlebell or a case of bottled water and use this to

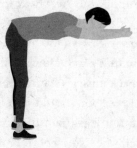

Hinge

add resistance to the exercise. Make sure you stop at your current end range of motion, or in other words, the point at which when you're lowering yourself you can no longer maintain a neutral spine position.

Sets/Reps: 3 Sets of 10 reps

Rest after the second exercise as needed. Shoot for thirty to ninety seconds.

1. Stand tall with your feet approximately shoulder width apart and toes pointing forward (slightly everted or out is okay if it feels more comfortable).
2. Place your hands on your hips and pull your shoulders straight back (retraction) as if you were trying to pinch something with your upper back.
3. Soften your knees very slightly and then make sure they do not travel any farther forward for the rest of the exercise.
4. Push your pelvis backward as if you were a tea kettle tipping water into a cup. Imagine that, as you're keeping your knees in that slightly bent position,

you are pushing your butt back toward an imaginary wall.

5. Make sure as you begin lowering yourself you keep your back in that pinched position so that your lats and other back muscles stay "turned on."

6. As you get lower, you should start to feel a stretch in the back of your legs (hamstrings/glutes).

7. Stop yourself when you feel you lose that tension or recognize that you are starting to "bend" forward without keeping a straight/neutral spine—at that point you've gone too far.

8. Stop yourself just before that position so that your posterior leg muscles stay engaged, push your pelvis forward slowly, maintain your back position, and stand back up squeezing your glutes or butt muscles at the top.

9. Repeat.

Single-Leg Dead Bug. The Dead Bug exercise does not require any additional equipment (you just need a soft, comfortable space to lie on your back), but when done correctly it serves as an incredibly efficient exercise to work your core!

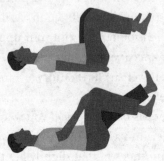

Single-leg dead bug

Pro Tip: To increase the degree of difficulty, try extending your opposing limbs simultaneously as opposed to doing just one leg at a time.

Sets/Reps: 3 Sets of 8 Reps on each leg

Rest after the second exercise as needed. Shoot for thirty to ninety seconds.

1. Lying on your back, with your arms palms down on the ground at forty-five degrees relative to your torso, bring your legs up so that they are bent at ninety degrees and are directly over top of your hips.
2. Engage and create tension in your core; when done effectively, your lower back will be pinned to the ground without any space.
3. Put your right arm on your right upper thigh/knee and, keeping your leg at ninety degrees, push backward hard into your hand to create further core tension.
4. Slowly extend your opposite leg while keeping your core tension everywhere else, slightly, and lightly tap your heel on the ground and then immediately return that leg to the starting position.
5. Do this for eight reps in a row (one leg at a time) then switch!

Biceps Curls. I find that if there's one exercise everyone likes to do, it's the bicep curl. Find some dumbbells, paint cans, water jugs, or even soup cans. It's time to curl!

Pro Tip: Change the orientation of your wrist to hit different sections of your biceps muscle, making sure you monitor and avoid any pain you notice.

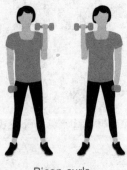

Bicep curls

Sets/Reps: 3 sets of 12 reps on each arm

1. Stand up straight with your feet about hip-width apart.
2. Hold your object balanced in your hand with your palm facing away from you and your arm extended/relaxed.
3. Keeping a straight back and resisting movement at your shoulder joint, bend at your elbow and begin curling the weight toward your shoulder.
4. Make sure your elbow stays in a mostly fixed position, your arms stay tight to your torso, and you're not using your back to help swing the weight upward.
5. Stop at about chest height, squeeze your bicep for about half a second, then slowly and with control lower back to the starting position and immediately begin again.
6. Repeat twelve times each side then switch arms.

Week 1, Day 4:
Cardiovascular Training/Flexibility

Since it's Week 1, we want to keep the difficulty to a manageable level. We want your rate of perceived exertion (RPE)—with 1 being little to no effort and 10 being all out—to be at about a 6 or a 7 today, so make adjustments to your effort accordingly.

Let's start with a 3:1 work-to-rest ratio, working hard for thirty seconds before dialing it back for ninety seconds of *active* rest and then repeating. For simplicity's sake, we will use running. Whether outside or on a treadmill, run or sprint at that RPE of 6 or 7 for thirty seconds before slowing down to a walk (not a complete stop). Use a phone, watch, or even count (slow enough) to make sure you're working and resting for the designated amount of time.

Pro Tip: Monitor your heart rate as you go if possible to find out what heart rate zones you were in and to help determine what substrates (proteins, fats, carbs) you were utilizing while you exercised!

Sets/Reps: 8 to 10 rounds of 30 seconds of work and 90 seconds of rest

Follow your workout with a couple of the stretches you learned on Day 2:

- Wall Hamstring Stretch
- Cat-Cow

End of week 1—congratulations! And let's keep going . . .

Weeks 2-4:
Resistance Training/Core/Balance

Your body adapts best when appropriate levels of volume, intensity, and resistance are practiced consistently over time. In other words, it's much smarter to stick with a training program for four, eight, or even twelve or more weeks depending on conditions rather than trying to do something new every time you work out. Yes, you'll get fatigued, but your body won't be able to make the strength, cardiovascular, muscular endurance, and mobility *progress* that I'm sure you all desire.

It also gives you time to master certain exercises and "own" movements until you're ready to progress to the next level of training. Make sure you give yourself the time to completely understand the exercises laid out for you and perform them with the proper form and level of difficulty.

Since this program is four weeks long, I'm going to explain how to progress yourself over the next three weeks until all four weeks are completed.

For your Resistance Training days, pick two exercises per workout to increase by one set. For example, say Week 1, Day 2 you choose Incline Push-Ups and Squats, Week 2, Day 2 would now have four sets of those exercises instead of three. Do the same for the following two weeks making sure to disperse the volume you add. In other words, you shouldn't include more than five sets of one exercise. Also, try to add 2.5 to 10 percent of the load you lift from week to week. For example, if you were able to squat with forty pounds, try adding an extra one to four pounds. For body weight exercises, try adding one or two reps week to week or slow down the tempo by an extra one to two seconds. By Week 4, your RPE should have gone from a 6 or a

7 to an 8 or a 9, which means you'll only have a couple of reps left in the tank with good form.

On the two separate Cardiovascular days, your progression techniques will focus on time, distance, and intensity. I recommend trying to add an additional five to ten minutes to your chosen exercise. For example, if you walked for thirty minutes Week 1, try to walk thirty-five or forty minutes Week 2. You can also add one or two intervals of work, decrease rest by five or ten seconds, or increase the exercise interval by five seconds, all with the goal of slightly increasing your "RPE" so that by Week 4, just like on the Resistance Training days, you're at an RPE of 7 or 8; meaning you could only do one or two more sprints before your form started breaking down.

For a free video demonstration of all exercises, visit www .webmd.com/takecontrol.

REFERENCES

Chapter One

American Diabetes Association. 2. Classification and diagnosis of diabetes: standards of medical care in diabetes—2020. *Diabetes Care.* 2020 Jan;43 (Suppl 1):S14–S31. doi: 10.2337/dc20-S002. PMID: 31862745.

Cheng YJ, Kanaya AM, Araneta MRG, Saydah SH, Kahn HS, Gregg EW, Fujimoto WY, Imperatore G. Prevalence of diabetes by race and ethnicity in the United States, 2011–2016. *JAMA.* 2019 Dec 24;322(24):2389–98. doi: 10.1001/jama.2019.19365. PMID: 31860047; PMCID: PMC6990660.

Grill V. LADA: A type of diabetes in its own right? *Curr Diabetes Rev.* 2019; 15(3):174–77. doi: 10.2174/1573399814666180716150905. PMID: 30009711.

Kleinberger JW, Pollin TI. Undiagnosed MODY: time for action. *Curr Diab Rep.* 2015 Dec;15(12):110. doi: 10.1007/s11892-015-0681-7. PMID: 26458381; PMCID: PMC4785020.

Viigimaa M, Sachinidis A, Toumpourleka M, Koutsampasopoulos K, Alliksoo S, Titma T. Macrovascular complications of type 2 diabetes mellitus. *Curr Vasc Pharmacol.* 2020;18(2):110–16. doi: 10.2174/1570161117666190405165151. PMID: 30961498.

Chapter Two

Cheng F, Carroll L, Joglekar MV, Januszewski AS, Wong KK, Hardikar AA, Jenkins AJ, Ma RCW. Diabetes, metabolic disease, and telomere length. *Lancet Diabetes Endocrinol.* 2021 Feb;9(2):117-126. doi: 10.1016/S2213-8587 (20)30365-X. Epub 2020 Nov 26. PMID: 33248477.

Cooper C, Sommerlad A, Lyketsos CG, Livingston G. Modifiable predictors of dementia in mild cognitive impairment: a systematic review and meta-analysis. *Am J Psychiatry.* 2015 Apr;172(4):323–34. doi: 10.1176/appi.ajp .2014.14070878. Epub 2015 Feb 20. PMID: 25698435.

Garfield V, Farmaki AE, Eastwood SV, Mathur R, Rentsch CT, Bhaskaran K, Smeeth L, Chaturvedi N. HbA1c and brain health across the entire glycaemic spectrum. *Diabetes Obes Metab.* 2021 Jan 19. doi: 10.1111/dom.14321. Epub ahead of print. PMID: 33464682.

Grandner MA, Seixas A, Shetty S, Shenoy S. Sleep duration and diabetes risk: population trends and potential mechanisms. *Curr Diab Rep.* 2016 Nov;16(11):106. doi: 10.1007/s11892-016-0805-8. PMID: 27664039; PMCID: PMC5070477.

Hunt HB, Miller NA, Hemmerling KJ, Koga M, Lopez KA, Taylor EA, Sellmeyer DE, Moseley KF, Donnelly E. Bone tissue composition in postmenopausal women varies with glycemic control from normal glucose tolerance to Type 2 diabetes mellitus. *J Bone Miner Res.* 2021 Feb;36(2): 334-346. doi: 10.1002/jbmr.4186. Epub 2020 Oct 29. PMID: 32970898.

Kumar M, Mishra L, Mohanty R, Nayak R. Diabetes and gum disease: the diabolic duo. *Diabetes Metab Syndr.* 2014 Oct–Dec;8(4):255–58. doi: 10.1016 /j.dsx.2014.09.022. Epub 2014 Oct 13. PMID: 25450824.

Moseley KF. Type 2 diabetes and bone fractures. *Curr Opin Endocrinol Diabetes Obes.* 2012 Apr;19(2):128–35. doi: 10.1097/MED.0b013e328350a6e1. PMID: 22262002; PMCID: PMC4753802.

Paul SK, Klein K, Thorsted BL, Wolden ML, Khunti K. Delay in treatment intensification increases the risks of cardiovascular events in patients with type 2 diabetes. *Cardiovasc Diabetol.* 2015 Aug 7;14:100. doi: 10.1186/s12933 -015-0260-x. PMID: 26249018; PMCID: PMC4528846.

Pourmemari MH, Shiri R. Diabetes as a risk factor for carpal tunnel syndrome: a systematic review and meta-analysis. *Diabet Med.* 2016 Jan;33(1): 10–16. doi: 10.1111/dme.12855. Epub 2015 Aug 18. PMID: 26173490.

Rayyan-Assi H, Feldman B, Leventer-Roberts M, Akriv A, Raz I. The relationship between inpatient hyperglycaemia and mortality is modified by baseline glycaemic status. *Diabetes Metab Res Rev.* 2020 Nov 2:e3420. doi: 10 .1002/dmrr.3420. Epub ahead of print. PMID: 33137237.

Zhao R, Wang Y, Fu T, Zhou W, Ge X, Sha X, Guo J, Dong C, Guo G. Gout and risk of diabetes mellitus: meta-analysis of observational studies. *Psychol Health Med.* 2020 Sep;25(8):917–30. doi: 10.1080/13548506.2019.1707241. Epub 2019 Dec 24. PMID: 31870181.

Chapter Three

Al-Mrabeh A, Hollingsworth KG, Shaw JAM, McConnachie A, Sattar N, Lean MEJ, Taylor R. 2-year remission of type 2 diabetes and pancreas morphology: a post-hoc analysis of the DiRECT open-label, cluster-randomised trial. *Lancet Diabetes Endocrinol.* 2020 Dec;8(12):939–48. doi: 10.1016/S2213 -8587(20)30303-X. Epub 2020 Oct 5. Erratum in: *Lancet Diabetes Endocrinol.* 2020 Dec;8(12):e7. PMID: 33031736.

Dutton GR, Lewis CE. The look AHEAD trial: implications for lifestyle intervention in type 2 diabetes mellitus. *Prog Cardiovasc Dis.* 2015 Jul–Aug; 58(1):69–75. doi: 10.1016/j.pcad.2015.04.002. Epub 2015 Apr 30. PMID: 25936906; PMCID: PMC4501472.

Eriksson KF, Lindgärde F. Prevention of type 2 (non-insulin-dependent) diabetes mellitus by diet and physical exercise. The 6-year Malmö feasibility study. *Diabetologia.* 1991 Dec;34(12):891–98. doi: 10.1007/BF00400196. PMID: 1778354.

le Roux CW, Astrup A, Fujioka K, Greenway F, Lau DCW, Van Gaal L, Ortiz RV, Wilding JPH, Skjøth TV, Manning LS, Pi-Sunyer X. SCALE Obesity Prediabetes NN8022-1839 Study Group. 3 years of liraglutide versus placebo for type 2 diabetes risk reduction and weight management in individuals with prediabetes: a randomised, double-blind trial. *Lancet.* 2017 Apr 8;389(10077):1399–1409. doi: 10.1016/S0140-6736(17)30069-7. Epub 2017 Feb 23. Erratum in: *Lancet.* 2017 Apr 8;389(10077):1398. PMID: 28237263.

Karter AJ, Nundy S, Parker MM, Moffet HH, Huang ES. Incidence of remission in adults with type 2 diabetes: the diabetes & aging study. *Diabetes Care.* 2014 Dec;37(12):3188–95. doi: 10.2337/dc14-0874. Epub 2014 Sep 17. PMID: 25231895; PMCID: PMC4237974.

Lean ME, Leslie WS, Barnes AC, Brosnahan N, Thom G, McCombie L, Peters C, Zhyzhneuskaya S, Al-Mrabeh A, Hollingsworth KG et al. Primary care-led weight management for remission of type 2 diabetes (DiRECT): an open-label, cluster-randomised trial. *Lancet.* 2018 Feb 10;391(10120):541–51. doi: 10.1016/S0140-6736(17)33102-1. Epub 2017 Dec 5. PMID: 29221645.

Perreault L, Kahn SE, Christophi CA, Knowler WC, Hamman RF; Diabetes Prevention Program Research Group. Regression from pre-diabetes to normal glucose regulation in the diabetes prevention program. *Diabetes Care.* 2009 Sep;32(9):1583–88. doi: 10.2337/dc09-0523. Epub 2009 Jul 8. PMID: 19587364; PMCID: PMC2732165.

Perreault L, Pan Q, Mather KJ, Watson KE, Hamman RF, Kahn SE. Diabetes Prevention Program Research Group. Effect of regression from prediabetes to normal glucose regulation on long-term reduction in diabetes risk: results from the Diabetes Prevention Program Outcomes Study. *Lancet.* 2012 Jun 16;379(9833):2243–51. doi: 10.1016/S0140-6736(12)60525-X. Epub 2012 Jun 9. PMID: 22683134; PMCID: PMC3555407.

Rooney MR, Rawlings AM, Pankow JS, et al. Risk of progression to diabetes among older adults with prediabetes. *JAMA Intern Med.* 2021;181(4):511–19. doi:10.1001/jamainternmed.2020.8774.

Sallar A, Dagogo-Jack S. Regression from prediabetes to normal glucose regulation: state of the science. *Exp Biol Med* (Maywood). 2020 May; 245(10):889–96. doi: 10.1177/1535370220915644. Epub 2020 Mar 25. PMID: 32212859; PMCID: PMC7268926.

Sampson M, Clark A, Bachmann M, et al. Lifestyle intervention with or without lay volunteers to prevent type 2 diabetes in people with impaired fasting glucose and/or nondiabetic hyperglycemia: a randomized clinical Trial. *JAMA Intern Med.* 2021;181(2):168–78. doi:10.1001/jamainternmed.2020.5938.

Tabák AG, Herder C, Rathmann W, Brunner EJ, Kivimäki M. Prediabetes: a high-risk state for diabetes development. *Lancet.* 2012;379(9833):2279–90. doi:10.1016/S0140-6736(12)60283-9.

Taylor R, Al-Mrabeh A, Zhyzhneuskaya S, Peters C, Barnes AC, Aribisala BS, Hollingsworth KG, Mathers JC, Sattar N, Lean MEJ. Remission of human type 2 diabetes requires decrease in liver and pancreas fat content but is dependent upon capacity for β cell recovery. *Cell Metab.* 2018 Oct 2;28(4): 547-556.e3. doi: 10.1016/j.cmet.2018.07.003. Epub 2018 Aug 2. Erratum in: *Cell Metab.* 2018 Oct 2;28(4):667. PMID: 30078554.

Wysham C, Shubrook J. Beta-cell failure in type 2 diabetes: mechanisms, markers, and clinical implications. *Postgrad Med.* 2020 Nov;132(8):676–86. doi: 10.1080/00325481.2020.1771047. Epub 2020 Jun 16. PMID: 32543261.

Chapter Four

Asnicar F, Berry SE, Valdes AM *et al.* Microbiome connections with host metabolism and habitual diet from 1,098 deeply phenotyped individuals. *Nat Med* 27, 321–332 (2021).

Bafeta A, Koh M, Riveros C, Ravaud P. Harms reporting in randomized controlled trials of interventions aimed at modifying microbiota: a systematic review. *Ann Intern Med.* 2018 Aug 21;169(4):240–247.

Bartkoski S, Day M. Alpha-lipoic acid for treatment of diabetic peripheral neuropathy. *Am Fam Physician.* 2016 May 1;93(9):786.

Cani PD, Amar J, Iglesias MA et al. Metabolic endotoxemia initiates obesity and insulin resistance. *Diabetes.* 2007 Jul;56(7):1761–72.

Chelakkot C, Choi Y, Kim DK et al. Akkermansia muciniphila-derived extracellular vesicles influence gut permeability through the regulation of tight junctions. *Exp Mol Med.* 2018; 50:e450.

Coates AM, Hill AM, Tan SY. Nuts and cardiovascular disease prevention. *Curr Atheroscler Rep.* 2018 Aug 9;20(10):48. doi: 10.1007/s11883-018-0749-3. PMID: 30094487.

d'Hennezel E, Abubucker S, Murphy LO, Cullen TW. Total lipopolysaccharide from the human gut microbiome silences toll-like receptor signaling. *mSystems.* 2017;2(6):e00046-17.

Díaz-Rizzolo DA, Serra A, Colungo C, Sala-Vila A, Sisó-Almirall A, Gomis R. Type 2 diabetes preventive effects with a 12-months sardine-enriched diet in elderly population with prediabetes: an interventional, randomized and controlled trial. *Clin Nutr.* 2021 May;40(5):2587–98. doi: 10.1016/j.clnu .2021.03.014. Epub 2021 Mar 18. PMID: 33932804.

Gijsbers L, Ding EL, Malik VS, de Goede J, Geleijnse JM, Soedamah-Muthu SS. Consumption of dairy foods and diabetes incidence: a dose-response meta-analysis of observational studies. *Am J Clin Nutr.* 2016 Apr;103(4):1111–24. doi: 10.3945/ajcn.115.123216. Epub 2016 Feb 24. PMID: 26912494.

Golbidi S, Badran M, Laher I. Diabetes and alpha lipoic acid. *Front Pharmacol.* 2011;2:69. Published 2011 Nov 17. doi:10.3389/fphar.2011.00069.

Gurung M, Li Z, You H et al. Role of gut microbiota in type 2 diabetes pathophysiology. *EBioMedicine.* 2020 Jan;51:102590.

Hartweg J, Perera R, Montori V et al., Farmer A. Omega-3 polyunsaturated fatty acids (PUFA) for type 2 diabetes mellitus. *Cochrane Database Syst Rev.* 2008 Jan 23;(1):CD003205.

Hasanzade F, Toliat M, Emami SA, Emamimoghaadam Z. The effect of cinnamon on glucose of type II diabetes patients. *J Tradit Complement Med.* 2013;3(3):171–74.

Hou YY, Ojo O, Wang LL, Wang Q, Jiang Q, Shao XY, Wang XH. A randomized controlled trial to compare the effect of peanuts and almonds on the cardio-metabolic and inflammatory parameters in patients with type 2 diabetes mellitus. *Nutrients.* 2018 Oct 23;10(11):1565. doi: 10.3390 /nu10111565. PMID: 30360498; PMCID: PMC6267433.

Kim Y, Keogh JB, Clifton PM. Benefits of nut consumption on insulin resistance and cardiovascular risk factors: multiple potential mechanisms of actions. *Nutrients.* 2017 Nov 22;9(11):1271. doi: 10.3390/nu9111271. PMID: 29165404; PMCID: PMC5707743.

Kinoshita M, Suzuki Y, Saito Y et al. Butyrate reduces colonic paracellular permeability by enhancing PPARgamma activation. *Biochem Biophys Res Commun.* 2002; 293:827–31.

Liu G, Zong G, Wu K, Hu Y, Li Y, Willett WC, Eisenberg DM, Hu FB, Sun Q. Meat cooking methods and risk of type 2 diabetes: results from three prospective cohort studies. *Diabetes Care.* 2018 May;41(5):1049–60. doi: 10.2337/dc17-1992. Epub 2018 Mar 12. PMID: 29530926; PMCID: PMC5911789.

Malik VS, Sun Q, van Dam RM, Rimm EB, Willett WC, Rosner B, Hu FB. Adolescent dairy product consumption and risk of type 2 diabetes in middle-aged women. *Am J Clin Nutr.* 2011 Sep;94(3):854–61. doi: 10.3945/ajcn.110.009621. Epub 2011 Jul 13. PMID: 21753066; PMCID: PMC3155931.

McMacken M, Shah S. A plant-based diet for the prevention and treatment of type 2 diabetes. *J Geriatr Cardiol.* 2017 May;14(5):342–54. doi: 10.11909/j.issn.1671-5411.2017.05.009. PMID: 28630614; PMCID: PMC5466941.

Mitri J, Muraru MD, Pittas AG. Vitamin D and type 2 diabetes: a systematic review. *Eur J Clin Nutr.* 2011 Sep;65(9):1005–15.

Schwingshackl L, Hoffmann G, Lampousi AM, Knüppel S, Iqbal K, Schwedhelm C, Bechthold A, Schlesinger S, Boeing H. Food groups and risk of type 2 diabetes mellitus: a systematic review and meta-analysis of prospective studies. *Eur J Epidemiol.* 2017 May;32(5):363–75. doi: 10.1007/s10654-017-0246-y. Epub 2017 Apr 10. PMID: 28397016; PMCID: PMC5506108.

Shan Z, Rehm CD, Rogers G, Ruan M, Wang DD, Hu FB, Mozaffarian D, Zhang FF, Bhupathiraju SN. Trends in dietary carbohydrate, protein, and fat intake and diet quality among US adults, 1999–2016. *JAMA.* 2019 Sep 24;322(12):1178–87. doi: 10.1001/jama.2019.13771. PMID: 31550032; PMCID: PMC6763999.

Suksomboon N, Poolsup N, Yuwanakorn A. Systematic review and meta-analysis of the efficacy and safety of chromium supplementation in diabetes. *J Clin Pharm Ther.* 2014 Jun;39(3):292–306.

Xu R, Zhang S, Tao A et al. Influence of vitamin E supplementation on glycaemic control: a meta-analysis of randomised controlled trials. *PLoS One.* 2014 Apr 16;9(4):e95008.

Zhang L, Qin Q, Liu M et al. Akkermansia muciniphila can reduce the damage of gluco/lipotoxicity, oxidative stress and inflammation, and normalize intestine microbiota in streptozotocin-induced diabetic rats. *Pathog Dis.* 2018 Jun 1;76(4).

Chapter Six

Church TS, Blair SN, Cocreham S, Johannsen N, Johnson W, Kramer K, Mikus CR, Myers V, Nauta M, Rodarte RQ, Sparks L, Thompson A, Earnest CP. Effects of aerobic and resistance training on hemoglobin A1c levels in patients with type 2 diabetes: a randomized controlled trial. *JAMA.* 2010 Nov 24;304(20):2253–62. doi: 10.1001/jama.2010.1710. Erratum in: JAMA. 2011 Mar 2;305(9):892. PMID: 21098771; PMCID: PMC3174102.

Colberg SR, Sigal RJ, Yardley JE, Riddell MC et al. Physical activity/exercise and diabetes: a position statement of the American Diabetes Association. *Diabetes Care.* 2016 Nov;39(11):2065–79.

Dijk JWV, Manders RJF, Tummers K, Bonomi AG et al. Both resistance- and endurance-type exercise reduce the prevalence of hyperglycemia in individuals with impaired glucose tolerance and in insulin-treated and non-insulin-treated type 2 diabetic patients. *Diabetologia.* 2012 May;55(5): 1273–82.

Eves ND, Plotnikoff RC. Resistance training and type 2 diabetes: considerations for implementation at the population level. *Diabetes Care.* 2006 Aug;29(8):1933–41. doi: 10.2337/dc05-1981. PMID: 16873809.

Francois ME, Little JP. Effectiveness and safety of high-intensity interval training in patients with type 2 diabetes. *Diabetes Spectr.* 2015 Jan;28(1): 39–44.

Galassetti P, Riddell MC. Exercise and type 1 diabetes (T1DM). *Compr Physiol.* 2013 Jul;3(3):1309–36. doi: 10.1002/cphy.c110040. PMID: 23897688.

Karstoft K, Winding K, Knudsen SH, et al. The effects of free-living interval-walking training on glycemic control, body composition, and physical fitness in type 2 diabetic patients: a randomized, controlled trial. *Diabetes Care* 2013;36:228–36.

Kirwan JP, Sacks J, Nieuwoudt S. The essential role of exercise in the management of type 2 diabetes. *Cleve Clin J Med.* 2017 Jul;84(7 Suppl 1):S15–S21. doi: 10.3949/ccjm.84.s1.03. PMID: 28708479; PMCID: PMC5846677.

Little JP, Gillen JB, Percival M, et al. Low-volume high-intensity interval training reduces hyperglycemia and increases muscle mitochondrial capacity in patients with type 2 diabetes. *J Appl Physiol* 2011;111:1554–60.

Mesinovic J, Zengin A, De Courten B et al. Sarcopenia and type 2 diabetes mellitus: a bidirectional relationship. *Diabetes Metab Syndr Obes.* 2019; 12:1057–72.

Olver TD, Laughlin MH. Endurance, interval sprint, and resistance exercise training: impact on microvascular dysfunction in type 2 diabetes. *Am J Physiol Heart Circ Physiol.* 2016 Feb 1;310(3):H337–50. doi: 10.1152/ajpheart .00440.2015. Epub 2015 Sep 25. PMID: 26408541; PMCID: PMC4796622.

Paffenbarger RS Jr, Lee I-M. Physical activity and fitness for health and longevity. *Res Q Exerc Sport* 1996;67:S11–S28.

Pan XR, Li GW, Hu YH, Wang JX et al. Effects of diet and exercise in preventing NIDDM in people with impaired glucose tolerance. The Da Qing IGT and Diabetes Study. *Diabetes Care.* 1997 Apr;20(4):537–44.

Shaban N, Kenno K, Milne K. The effects of a 2 week modified high intensity interval training program on the homeostatic model of insulin resistance (HOMA-IR) in adults with type 2 diabetes. *J Sports Medicine Phys Fitness* 2014;54:203–9.

Stensvold D, Viken H, Steinshamn SL et al. Effect of exercise training for five years on all cause mortality in older adults—the Generation 100 study: randomized controlled trial. *BMJ.* 2020 Oct 7;371m3485.

Weston KS, Wisløff U, Coombes JS. High-intensity interval training in patients with lifestyle-induced cardiometabolic disease: a systematic review and meta-analysis. *Brit J Sports Med* 2014;48:1227–34.

Chapter Seven

Asuzu CC, Walker RJ, Williams JS, Egede LE. Pathways for the relationship between diabetes distress, depression, fatalism and glycemic control in adults with type 2 diabetes. *J Diabetes Complications.* 2017 Jan;31(1):169–74. doi: 10.1016/j.jdiacomp.2016.09.013. Epub 2016 Sep 30. PMID: 27746088; PMCID: PMC5209296.

Bădescu SV, Tătaru C, Kobylinska L, Georgescu EL, Zahiu DM, Zăgrean AM, Zăgrean L. The association between diabetes mellitus and depression. *J Med Life.* 2016 Apr–Jun;9(2):120–25. PMID: 27453739; PMCID: PMC4863499.

Brieler JA, Lustman PJ, Scherrer JF, Salas J, Schneider FD. Antidepressant medication use and glycaemic control in co-morbid type 2 diabetes and depression. *Fam Pract.* 2016 Feb;33(1):30–36. doi: 10.1093/fampra/cmv100. Epub 2016 Jan 7. PMID: 26743722.

Brown LC, Majumdar SR, Newman SC, Johnson JA. History of depression increases risk of type 2 diabetes in younger adults. *Diabetes Care.* 2005;28(5):1063-7.

Dennick K, Sturt J, Speight J. What is diabetes distress and how can we measure it? A narrative review and conceptual model. *J Diabetes Complications.* 2017 May;31(5):898–911. doi: 10.1016/j.jdiacomp.2016.12.018. Epub 2017 Feb 14. PMID: 28274681.

Fisher L, Polonsky WH, Hessler D. Addressing diabetes distress in clinical care: a practical guide. *Diabet Med.* 2019 Jul;36(7):803–12. doi: 10.1111/dme.13967. Epub 2019 May 7. PMID: 30985025.

Gonzalez JS, Shreck E, Psaros C, Safren SA. Distress and type 2 diabetes-treatment adherence: A mediating role for perceived control. *Health Psychol.* 2015 May;34(5):505–13. doi: 10.1037/hea0000131. Epub 2014 Aug 11. PMID: 25110840; PMCID: PMC4324372.

Hirosaki M, Ohira T, Kajiura M, Kiyama M, Kitamura A, Sato S, Iso H. Effects of a laughter and exercise program on physiological and psychological health among community-dwelling elderly in Japan: randomized controlled trial. *Geriatr Gerontol Int.* 2013 Jan;13(1):152–60. doi: 10.1111/j.1447-0594.2012.00877.x. Epub 2012 Jun.

Holt RI, de Groot M, Golden SH. Diabetes and depression. *Curr Diab Rep.* 2014 Jun;14(6):491. doi: 10.1007/s11892-014-0491-3. PMID: 24743941; PMCID: PMC4476048.

Joseph JJ, Golden SH. Cortisol dysregulation: the bidirectional link between stress, depression, and type 2 diabetes mellitus. *Ann N Y Acad Sci.* 2017 Mar;1391(1):20–34. doi: 10.1111/nyas.13217. Epub 2016 Oct 17. PMID: 27750377; PMCID: PMC5334212.

Kalra S, Verma K, Singh Balhara YP. Management of diabetes distress. *J Pak Med Assoc.* 2017 Oct;67(10):1625–27. PMID: 28955090.

Mora P, Buskirk A, Lyden M, Parkin CG, Borsa L, Petersen B. Use of a novel, remotely connected diabetes management system is associated with increased treatment satisfaction, reduced diabetes distress, and improved glycemic control in individuals with insulin-treated diabetes: first results from the Personal Diabetes Management Study. *Diabetes Technol Ther.* 2017

Dec;19(12):715–22. doi: 10.1089/dia.2017.0206. Epub 2017 Oct 13. PMID: 29027812; PMCID: PMC5734194.

Owens-Gary MD, Zhang X, Jawanda S, Bullard KM, Allweiss P, Smith BD. The importance of addressing depression and diabetes distress in adults with type 2 diabetes. *J Gen Intern Med.* 2019 Feb;34(2):320–24. doi: 10.1007/s11606-018-4705-2. Epub 2018 Oct 22. PMID: 30350030; PMCID: PMC6374277.

Perrin NE, Davies MJ, Robertson N, Snoek FJ, Khunti K. The prevalence of diabetes-specific emotional distress in people with type 2 diabetes: a systematic review and meta-analysis. *Diabet Med.* 2017 Nov;34(11):1508–20. doi: 10.1111/dme.13448. Epub 2017 Aug 31. PMID: 28799294.

Polonsky WH, Layne JE, Parkin CG, Kusiak CM, Barleen NA, Miller DP, Zisser H, Dixon RF. Impact of participation in a virtual diabetes clinic on diabetes-related distress in individuals with type 2 diabetes. *Clin Diabetes.* 2020 Oct;38(4):357–62. doi: 10.2337/cd19-0105. PMID: 33132505; PMCID: PMC7566922.

Schmitt A, Reimer A, Kulzer B, Haak T, Ehrmann D, Hermanns N. How to assess diabetes distress: comparison of the Problem Areas in Diabetes Scale (PAID) and the Diabetes Distress Scale (DDS). *Diabet Med.* 2016 Jun; 33(6):835–43. doi: 10.1111/dme.12887. Epub 2015 Sep 8. PMID: 26287511.

Semenkovich K, Brown ME, Svrakic DM, Lustman PJ. Depression in type 2 diabetes mellitus: prevalence, impact, and treatment. *Drugs.* 2015 Apr; 75(6):577–87. doi: 10.1007/s40265-015-0347-4. PMID: 25851098.

Sharma VK, Singh TG. Chronic stress and diabetes mellitus: interwoven pathologies. *Curr Diabetes Rev.* 2020;16(6):546–56. doi: 10.2174/1573399815666191111152248. PMID: 31713487.

Snoek FJ, Bremmer MA, Hermanns N. Constructs of depression and distress in diabetes: time for an appraisal. *Lancet Diabetes Endocrinol.* 2015 Jun;3(6):450–60. doi: 10.1016/S2213-8587(15)00135-7. Epub 2015 May 17. PMID: 25995123.

Watson K, Nasca C, Aasly L, McEwen B, Rasgon N. Insulin resistance, an unmasked culprit in depressive disorders: promises for interventions. *Neuropharmacology.* 2018 Jul 1;136(Pt B):327–334. doi: 10.1016/j.neuropharm.2017.11.038. Epub 2017 Nov 26. PMID: 29180223.

Watson KT, Simard JF, Henderson VW, Nutkiewicz L, Lamers F, Rasgon N, Penninx B. Association of insulin resistance with depression severity and remission status: defining a metabolic endophenotype of depression. *JAMA*

Psychiatry. 2020 Dec 2:e203669. doi: 10.1001/jamapsychiatry.2020.3669. Epub ahead of print. PMID: 33263725; PMCID: PMC7711568.

Zander-Schellenberg T, Collins IM, Miché M, Guttmann C, Lieb R, Wahl K. Does laughing have a stress-buffering effect in daily life? An intensive longitudinal study. *PLoS One*. 2020 Jul 9;15(7):e0235851. doi: 10.1371 /journal.pone.0235851. PMID: 32645063; PMCID: PMC7347187.

Chapter Eight

Anothaisintawee T, Reutrakul S, Van Cauter E, Thakkinstian A. Sleep disturbances compared to traditional risk factors for diabetes development: systematic review and meta-analysis. *Sleep Med Rev*. 2015;30:11–24.

Charles LE, Gu JK, Andrew ME, Violanti JM et al. Sleep duration and biomarkers of metabolic function among police officers. *J Occup Environ Med*. 2011;53(8):831–37.

Curtis DS, Fuller-Rowell TE, El-Sheikh M, Carnethon M et al. Habitual sleep as a contributor to racial differences in cardiometabolic risk. *Proc Natl Acad Sci USA*. 2017 Aug 15;114(33):8889–94.

Doumit J, Prasad B. Sleep apnea in type 2 diabetes. *Diabetes Spect*. 2016 Feb;29(1):14–19.

Duncan BB, Schmidt MI, Pankow JS et al. Low-grade systemic inflammation and the development of type 2 diabetes: the atherosclerosis risk in communities study. *Diabetes*. 2003 Jul;52(7):1799–1805.

Grandner MA, Williams NJ, Knutson KL, Roberts D, Jean-Louis G. Sleep disparity, race/ethnicity, and socioeconomic position. *Sleep Med*. 2016 Feb; 18:7–18.

Haack M, Sanchez E, Mullington JM. Elevated inflammatory markers in response to prolonged sleep restriction are associated with increased pain experience in healthy volunteers. *Sleep*. 2007 Sep; 30(9):1145–52.

Hackett RA, Kivimaki M, Kumari M, Steptoe A. Diurnal cortisol patterns, future diabetes, and impaired glucose metabolism in the Whitehall II Cohort Study. *J Clin Endocrinol Metab*. 2016 Feb; 101(2):619–25.

Mani KM, Shankar K, Zigman JM. Ghrelin's relationship to blood glucose. *Endocrinology*. 2019 May 1;160(5):1247–61.

Meek TH, Morton GJ. Leptin, diabetes, and the brain. *Indian J Endocrinol Metab*. 2012 Dec; 16(Suppl 3):S534–S42.

Office of Disease Prevention and Health Promotion. *Healthy People 2030 objective topic areas.* US Department of Health and Human Services; Washington: 2020. https://health.gov/healthypeople.

Omisade A, Buxton OM, Rusak B. Impact of acute sleep restriction on cortisol and leptin levels in young women. *Physiol Behav.* 2010 Apr 19.

Patel SR, Zhu X, Storfer-Isser A, Mehra R, Jenny NS, Tracy R, et al. Sleep duration and biomarkers of inflammation. *Sleep.* 2009;32(2):200–4.

Spiegel K, Leproult R, Cauter EV. Impact of sleep debt on metabolic and endocrine function. *Lancet.* 1999 Oct 23; 354(9188):1435–39.

Spiegel K, Tasali E, Penev P, Van Cauter E. Brief communication: sleep curtailment in healthy young men is associated with decreased leptin levels, elevated ghrelin levels, and increased hunger and appetite. *Ann Intern Med.* 2004;141(11):846–50.

Tan E, Scott EM. Circadian rhythms, insulin action, and glucose homeostasis. *Curr Opin Clin Nutr Metab Care.* 2014 Jul; 17(4):343–48.

Zizi F, Pandey A, Murray-Bachmann R, Vincent M et al. Race/ethnicity, sleep duration, and diabetes mellitus: analysis of the National Health Interview Survey. *Am J Med.* 2012 Feb;125(2):162–67.

Chapter Nine

Aune D, Hartaigh BO, Vatten LJ. Resting heart rate and the risk of type 2 diabetes: A systematic review and dose-response meta-analysis of cohort studies. *Nutr Metab Cardiovasc Dis.* 2015 Jun;25(6):526–34.

Chiodini I, Adda G, Scillitani A, Coletti F et al. Cortisol secretion in patients with type 2 diabetes: relationship with chronic complications. *Diabetes Care.* 2007 Jan;30(1):83–88.

Dias JP, Joseph JJ, Kluwe B, Zhao S et al. The longitudinal association of changes in diurnal cortisol features with fasting glucose: MESA. *Psychoneuroendocrinology.* 2020 Sep;119:104698.

Emdin CA, Anderson SG, Woodward M, Rahimi K. Usual blood pressure and risk of new-onset diabetes: evidence from 4.1 million adults and a meta-analysis of prospective studies. *J Am Coll Cardiol.* 2015 Oct 6;66(14): 1552–62.

Geer EB, Islam J, Buettner C. Mechanisms of glucocorticoid-induced insulin resistance. *Endocrinol Metab Clin North Am.* 2014 Mar; 43(1):75–102.

Hackett RA, Kivimaki M, Kumari M, Steptoe A. Diurnal cortisol patterns, future diabetes, and impaired glucose metabolism in the Whitehall II Cohort Study. *J Clin Endocrinol Metab.* 2016 Feb; 101(2):619–25.

Hackett RA, Steptoe A. Type 2 diabetes mellitus and psychological stress—a modifiable risk factor. *Nat Rev Endocrinol.* 2017 Sep;13(9):547–60.

Kramer CK, Mehmood S, Suen RS. Dog ownership and survival: a systematic review and meta-analysis. *Circ Cardiovasc Qual Outcomes.* 2019 Oct;12(10):e005554. doi: 10.1161/CIRCOUTCOMES.119.005554. Epub 2019 Oct 8. PMID: 31592726.

Li J, Jarczok MN, Loerbroks A, Schollgen I et al. Work stress is associated with diabetes and prediabetes: cross-sectional results from the MIPH Cohort Studies. *Int J Behav Med.* 2013 Dec;20(4):495–503.

Linnemann A, Ditzen B, Strahler J, Doerr JM, Nater UM. Music listening as a means of stress reduction in daily life. *Psychoneuroendocrinology.* 2015 Oct;60:82–90. doi: 10.1016/j.psyneuen.2015.06.008. Epub 2015 Jun 21. PMID: 26142566.

Lloyd C, Smith J, Weinger K. Stress and diabetes: a review of the links. *Diabetes Spectrum.* 2005 Apr; 18(2):121–27.

Mooy JM, Vries HD, Grootenhuis PA, Bouter LM et al. Major stressful life events in relation to prevalence of undetected type 2 diabetes: the Hoorn Study. *Diabetes Care.* 2000 Feb;23(2):197–201.

Morey, JN, Boggero IA, Scott AB, Segerstrom SC. Current directions in stress and human immune function. *Curr Opin Psychol.* 2015 Oct 1; 5:13–17.

Smith EN, Young MD, Crum AJ. Stress, mindsets, and success in Navy SEALs special warfare training. *Front Psychol.* 2020 Jan 15;10:2962. doi: 10.3389 /fpsyg.2019.02962. PMID: 32010023; PMCID: PMC6974804.

Williams ED, Magliano DJ, Tapp RJ, Oldenburg BF et al. Psychosocial stress predicts abnormal glucose metabolism: the Australian Diabetes, Obesity and Lifestyle (AusDiab) study. *Ann Behav Med.* 2013 Aug;46(1):62–72.

Zamani-Alavijeh, F., Araban, M., Koohestani, H.R. et al. The effectiveness of stress management training on blood glucose control in patients with type 2 diabetes. *Diabetol Metab Syndr* 10, 39 (2018).

INDEX

ABOUT THE AUTHOR

JOHN WHYTE, MD, MPH, is a popular physician and writer who has been communicating to the public about health issues for nearly two decades.

In his role as chief medical officer of WebMD, Dr. Whyte leads efforts to develop and expand strategic partnerships that create meaningful change around important and timely public health issues. Before joining WebMD, Whyte served as the director of professional affairs and stakeholder engagement at the Center for Drug Evaluation and Research at the US Food and Drug Administration. Dr. Whyte worked with health care professionals, patients, and patient advocates, providing them with a focal point for advocacy, enhanced two-way communication, and collaboration, assisting them in navigating the FDA on issues concerning drug development, review, and drug safety. He also developed numerous initiatives to address diversity in clinical trials.

Dr. Whyte worked for nearly a decade as the chief medical expert and vice president, health and medical education, at Discovery Channel, the leading nonfiction television network. In this role, he developed, designed, and delivered educational programming that appealed to medical and lay audiences. This included television shows and online content that won more than fifty awards, including numerous Tellys, CINE Golden Eagles, and Freddies.

Whyte is a board-certified internist. He completed an internal medicine residency at Duke University Medical Center and earned a master of public health in health policy and management at Harvard University School of Public Health. Before arriving in Washington, DC, he was a health services research fellow at Stanford and attending physician in the department of medicine.